APPLICATIONS OF LASERS AND LASER SYSTEMS

David Beach

Allen Shotwell

Paul Essue

PTR Prentice Hall, Englewood Cliffs, New Jersey 07632

Library of Congress Cataloging-in-Publication Data

Beach, David P.
Applications of lasers and laser systems / by David Beach, Allen Shotwell, Paul Essue.
p. cm.
Includes index.
ISBN 0-13-041930-3
1. Lasers. I. Shotwell, Allen. II. Essue, PAul, III. Title
TA1675.B42 1993
621.36'6--dc20 93-14847
CIP

Editorial production: *bookworks*
Acquisitions Editor: *Karen Gettman*
Cover designer: *Greg Wilkin*
Buyer: *Mary Elizabeth McCartney*

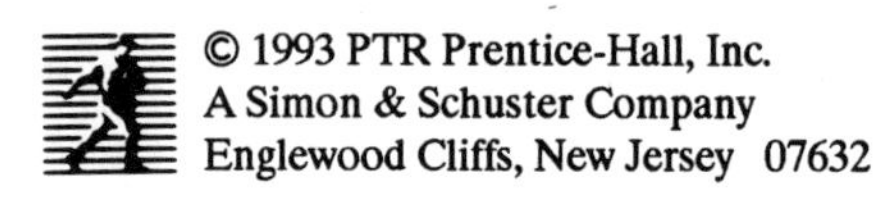

A Simon & Schuster Company
Englewood Cliffs, New Jersey 07632

The publisher offers discounts on this book when ordered in bulk quantities. For more information contact:

Corporate Sales Department
PTR Prentice Hall
113 Sylvan Avenue
Englewood Cliffs, New Jersey 07632

Phone: 201-592-2863
FAX: 201-592-2249

Printed in the United States of America

10 9 8 7 6 5 4 3 2 1

ISBN 0-13-041930-3

Prentice-Hall International (UK) Limited, *London*
Prentice-Hall of Australia Pty. Limited, *Sydney*
Prentice-Hall Canada Inc., *Toronto*
Prentice-Hall Hispanoamericana, S.A., *Mexico*
Prentice-Hall of India Private Limited, *New Delhi*
Prentice-Hall of Japan, Inc., *Tokyo*
Simon & Schuster Asia Pte. Ltd., *Singapore*
Editora Prentice-Hall do Brasil, Ltda., *Rio de Janeiro*

To my wife,
Ethel
D.B.

To my dad,
Hugh
A.S.

CONTENTS

PREFACE

About This Book

The information contained in this book is divided into three major areas. Unit I provides the reader with background information on lasers, beginning with the fundamentals of how a laser works (Chapter 1) and extending through the common laser types, optics, and major components of laser systems. Unit II provides a general discussion of common laser applications. Each chapter includes information on typical lasers used in the application, factors to be considered and actual examples of applications. The final unit (Unit III) gives guidelines for troubleshooting, maintaining, and installing common laser systems.

The reader's approach to this book should depend on his or her own level of understanding, and the specific information required. Although it is possible to read the book by following a natural progression beginning with Chapter 1 and following through sequentially, it may be more useful to pick a starting point that fits your particular situation. For example, a reader new to the laser field would want to begin with Unit I to gain the background necessary for understanding the topics in the rest of the book. A reader who already has a grasp of lasers, but is interested in a particular application would turn to Unit II, and a reader with knowledge of lasers who is presented with a specific problem in troubleshooting or maintenance would start with Unit III. The choice of starting points should not limit the reader to a particular unit. Sometimes, it is necessary to skip to another unit to expand upon a particular topic. For facilitating the process, each unit begins with a guide to the information that it contains—so you can pinpoint where it may be best to begin.

Acknowledgements

The authors would like to extend special thanks to Colin Payne, Manager of Technical Support and Marketing — *Coherent General, Inc.*, for his significant contribution toward the preparation of the troubleshooting procedures that are included in Unit III. Appreciation is also extended to Karen C. Ronning, Senior Technical Writer — *Electro Scientific Industries*, and Reuben E. Nystrom, Manager of Advertising & Training — *Cincinnati Incorporated*, for their contributions toward the development of this manuscript.

Unit I

FUNDAMENTALS OF LASERS

The laser in theory and construction combines the principles of several disciplines. In theory, the laser is based on physics and electronics. In construction, it incorporates electronics, optics, chemistry and even fluids. With such a variety of information, a discussion of laser fundamentals could easily fill several books. In fact many excellent books have been written on the topics discussed in this unit, and the reader is encouraged to make use of the bibliographies at the end of each chapter.

Unit I tries to provide a reasonably complete discussion of laser fundamentals in a limited space. Topics in Unit I are meant as a review or introduction that facilitates an understanding of the other two units. Chapter 1 introduces the theory of the laser and some of the physics it involves in an essentially non-mathematical discussion. The beginning of the chapter also provides a summary of this information for a quick review or introduction.

Chapter 2 provides information on some of the most common types of lasers. Basic principles of operation, common designs and beam characteristics are given for the Nd:YAG, CO_2, argon, ruby, dye and semiconductor laser.

The principles of geometrical and wave optics are discussed in Chapter 3. The main phenomena involving these areas are covered along with some information on common calculations. The topic of quantum optics is left to the discussions in Chapter 1.

Since the laser itself is supported by an array of other devices, Chapter 4 covers them under the general heading of laser systems. Included are scanners, modulators, detectors, positioning systems, and optical components. These devices are also referred to and discussed in later chapters.

Please remember that lasers are hazardous devices, and the appropriate safety procedures and cautions should be well understood before any work is done with them. Appendix C provides a discussion of laser safety and should be read carefully before venturing into the lab or shop where a laser is used.

1

INTRODUCTION TO LASERS

Introduction

Light Amplification by Stimulated Emission of Radiation describes a wide range of devices. There are many different types of lasers, but they all share a basic element; each contains a material capable of amplifying radiation. The physical principle responsible for this amplification is called stimulated emission.

The laser has had a tremendous impact on various fields in science and technology and is a device that seems to have unlimited applications. It has practically revolutionized the fields of optical technology and spectroscopy, and is now being used in a wide variety of applications in industry. Lasers are now used extensively in medicine, communications, national defense, measurement, and as a precise light source in many scientific investigations. Many types of lasers are commercially available with a large range of output wavelengths and powers.

In 1917, Albert Einstein developed the concept of stimulated emission, the phenomenon that is utilized in lasers. Stimulated emission produces amplification of light so that the buildup of high-intensity light in the laser can occur. Laser light was found to have significantly different characteristics from ordinary light sources. It was these characteristics, notably its intensity, and directivity, which allowed the laser to find so many practical applications. Typical applications of industrial lasers such as the Nd:YAG and the CO_2 are cutting, drilling, and welding.

An understanding of laser technology should be preceded by a basic comprehension of the principles and theory of laser operation. This chapter is a broad introduction to lasers by presenting their essential principles, properties, and characteristics.

1.1 An Overview of Laser Technology

1.1.1 The Laser

Basically, a laser consists of a cavity, with mirrors at the ends, filled with lasable material. Just as a home stereo system is a sound amplifier, a laser system is a light amplifier.

1.1.2 Reasons for Using a Laser

Some of the reasons for using lasers include: (i) the process may be significantly less expensive than other techniques; (ii) it may be difficult or impossible to complete the task any other way; (iii) the laser cutting edge does not get dull; and (iv) the laser can be computer-controlled to achieve reliable production.

1.1.3 Laser Material

Lasers are available in all three states of matter: solid, liquid, and gas. Some examples of solids are ruby, YAG, and glass lasers. Solid lasers are also called solid-state. Examples of gas lasers are helium-neon, argon, excimer, xenon, and carbon dioxide. Liquid lasers are generally dye lasers.

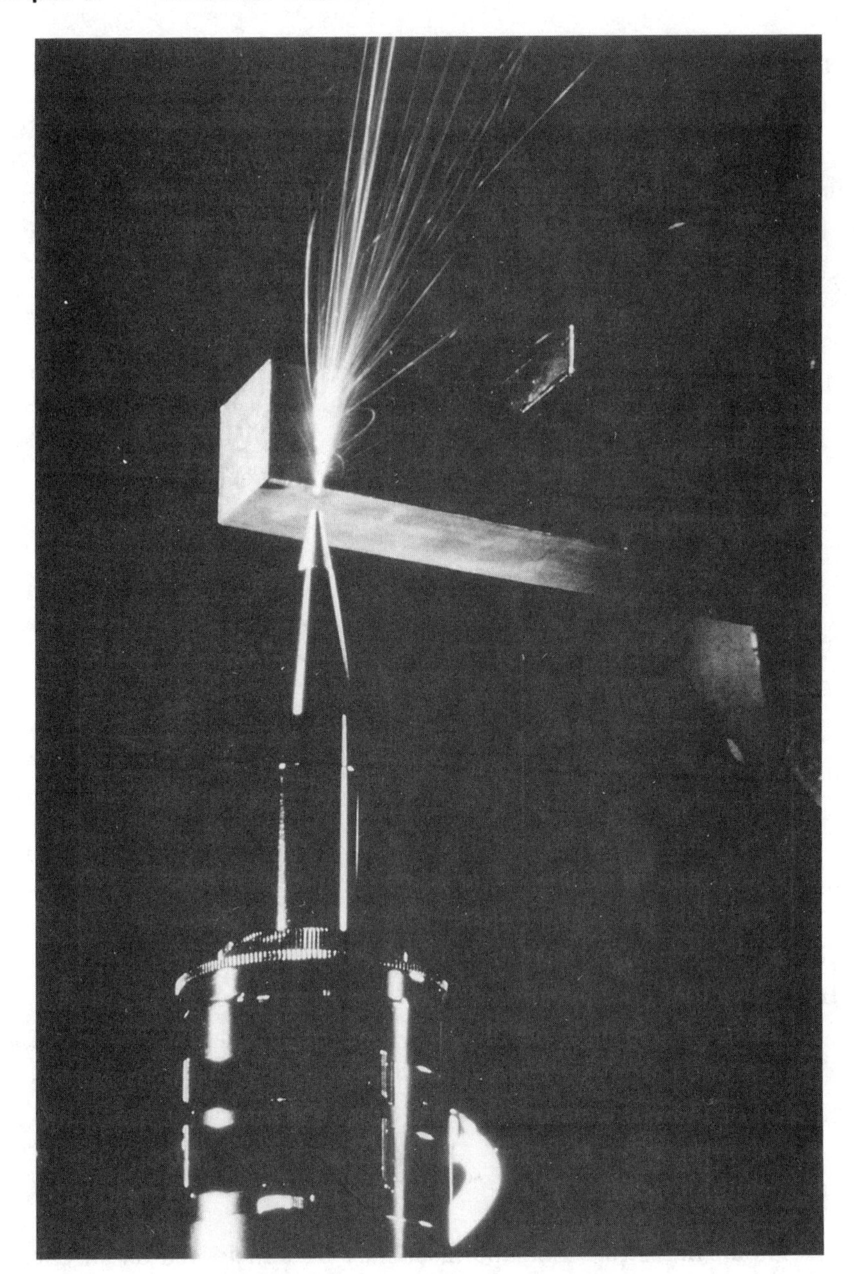

Figure 1-1 Laser beam cutting through metal
(Courtesy of Coherent General, Inc.)

1.1.4 Laser Colors

A particular laser has its own characteristic color. For example, ruby is red, YAG is invisible infrared, argon is green, CO_2 lasers emit in the far infrared, and excimers are ultraviolet. Lasers span the entire light spectrum from infrared to ultraviolet.

1.1.5 Laser System

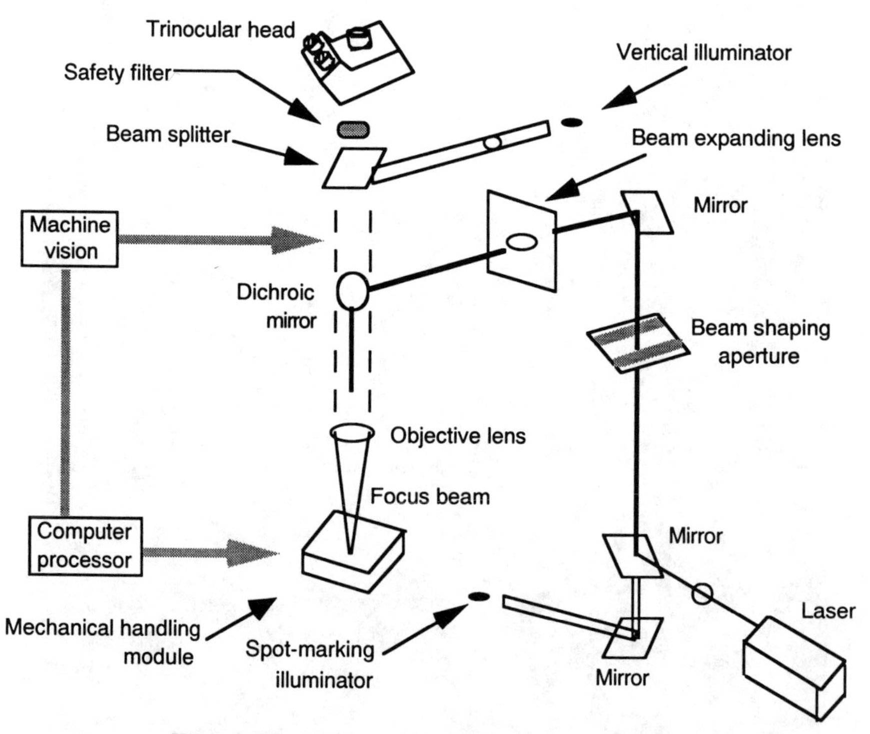

Figure 1-2 Optical schematic of an industrial laser

As an industrial tool, the laser may be considered as an energy source. For applications involving drilling or cutting, the laser beam is directed through a lens to concentrate the beam. Directing the beam on a material to be drilled, cut, or welded converts the laser energy into heat that can vaporize or melt the material. A complete industrial laser usually consists of the laser unit, an optical system (to shape, direct, and focus the beam), a mechanical part's handler (usually robotic), computer controller, and a machine vision system. Figure 1-2 shows how a typical system might be arranged.

1.1.6 Laser Power

Lasers provide a wide range of output power—from milliwatts, to tens of thousands of watts. Power is the rate of doing work in units of watts, and indicates the "strength" of a laser beam. A watt is one joule of energy per second. A 100-watt light bulb and a 100-watt continuous wave laser both emit 100 joules of energy every second. The difference between the two sources is that the bulb puts the light out in all different directions while the laser's light comes out in a beam. Even one millijoule (0.001 J) of light concentrated in a spot of 0.001 inch achieves an energy density of 640 joules per square inch. If this 0.001 joule is in a laser pulse of half a microsecond (0.0000005 second) duration, the power is 2,000 watts in a 0.001-inch spot. The focused power density is now over one billion watts per square inch! Such highly concentrated power is how lasers vaporize material.

1.1.7 Continuous Wave Laser

Some lasers emit continuously (cw) while others are pulsed—a cw laser emits a steady stream of light while pulsed lasers emit light in short spurts. Laser hole drillers are pulsed while laser welders can be cw for seam welds or pulsed for spot welds. Lasers used in light shows are cw and so are the common red helium-neon lasers used in supermarket scanners. YAG lasers may be operated cw or pulsed. Xenon lasers are always pulsed.

1.1.8 The Source of Excitation Energy

To generate a laser beam, it is necessary to redistribute the amount of atoms that normally exist in certain atomic energy levels of the laser medium. This requires an external source of excitation energy called the "pump energy." In gas and semiconductor lasers, the excitation mechanism may consist of an electrical-current flow through the active medium. Solid and liquid lasers often use optical pumps.

Optical Pumping. Most solid-state and dye lasers are optically pumped, meaning that the energy source is light. Flash lamps are used for pulsed YAG lasers and arc lamps for cw YAG lasers. Krypton gas is used in the lamps because the particular color emitted by krypton is readily absorbed by the neodymium in the YAG.

Electrical Pumping. Gas lasers are usually excited by a gas discharge. For example, argon is an electrically pumped ion gas laser. The active medium is ionized argon. Argon lasers emit mostly in the blue-green region of the spectrum. A high-voltage trigger mechanism initiates ionization in an ion laser. A gas discharge follows ionization, driven by a capacitor discharge.

1.1.9 Wavelength

A wavelength is the length or distance between the peaks of the light wave. Green light has a wavelength of 0.5 micron (a micron is a millionth of a meter and is abbreviated 1×10^{-6} meter). Blue light has a wavelength of 0.4 micron, and the wavelength for red light is 0.7 micron. Laser light is available in all colors from red to violet, as well as outside the limits of the conventional optical spectrum. Some of the available laser light is "tunable," which means that certain lasers have the property of emitting light at some chosen wavelength within a range of wavelengths.

1.1.10 Photon Energy

A photon is a quantum of light having a characteristic wavelength and energy content. Its energy and wavelength are related, and the photon's energy depends on the energy of the atom that emits it.

1.1.11 The Laser Medium

This is also referred to as the active medium and consists of a collection of atoms or molecules that can be excited to a state of inverted population, which is the state where more atoms are in an excited state than in some lower energy state. The laser medium may be a solid, liquid, gas, or junction between two semiconductor materials. It can be thought of as an optical amplifier that is capable of sustaining stimulated emission because of its atomic structure.

1.1.12 Spontaneous Emission

The atoms or molecules in the laser medium are excited by the pumping source. Excited atoms, which contain more energy than atoms in the ground state, will only remain excited for a short period of time. Eventually the atom (or molecule) will release its extra energy (usually as a photon of light) and return to its ground state. This type of release of light energy is known as *spontaneous emission.*

1.1.13 Stimulated Emission of Radiation

If an excited atom collides with one of the spontaneously emitted photons, this atom is caused (stimulated) to make its quantum leap or transition toward the ground state. In so doing, the atom emits two photons; the one that came in plus the one from the transition. This is *stimulated emission* (one photon into the atom, two out). In spontaneous emission, there are no photons in, but one out. Figure 1-3 illustrates the two processes.

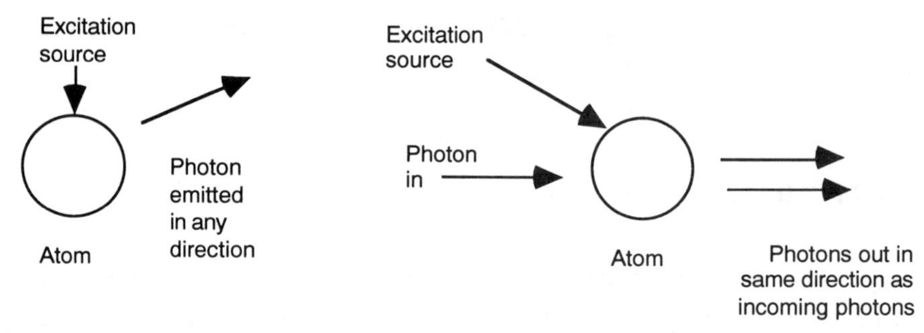

Figure 1-3(a) Spontaneous emission **Figure 1-3(b)** Stimulated emission

1.1.14 Laser Beam

The two photons coming out of a stimulated emission travel in the same direction as the one that came in. If two photons going south strike two more excited atoms, now there will be four photons going south. If these four photons strike four more excited atoms, then there are eight, then 16, 32, etc., all with the characteristic laser wavelength. This chain reaction explains, at the atomic level, how the laser amplifies light (amplification). It is also one of the reasons why laser light travels only in one direction (directivity).

1.1.15 Laser Mirrors

A simplified reason for laser light appearing in a beam is because every laser has at least two end mirrors. One mirror is almost 100% reflective so most of the beam reflects from it and back into the laser medium, for amplification. The other mirror is only partially reflective. Some of the beam reflects back into the laser and some passes through the mirror. The laser output portion that comes out of the partial reflecting mirror is the usable laser beam. The beam goes both ways between the mirrors but only one way outside. Within the mirrors the beam is said to oscillate.

1.1.16 Optical Components

Optical components (other than the laser mirrors) are needed to manipulate the beam so it can be used in various applications. Optics are used to reflect (mirrors) and refract or focus (lenses) light. They are also used for wavelength selection, altering polarizing components of light, and breaking up light into its spectral components. These are considered "passive" optical functions, because the components do not require any special control or input power to perform them. Active components operate under active control or need input power to perform their functions. Active components include modulators, which alter beam intensity, and scanners that move a beam.

1.2 General Properties of Light

1.2.1 Electromagnetic Radiation

The light emitted by a laser is electromagnetic radiation (e.m). The term e.m radiation includes a continuous range of many types of radiation. Electromagnetic radiation is said to have a wave nature that consists of vibrating electric and magnetic fields. A wave is a disturbance that transmits energy from one point to another. Waves can be characterized by their frequency, i.e., the number of cycles per second of oscillation of the electric or magnetic field. The length over which the wave repeats itself is the wavelength, i.e., the distance between the peaks of a wave.

Wave motion propagates with a characteristic velocity c (taken to be the velocity of light or 3×10^{10} cm per second). In all portions of the optical spectrum, shown in Figure 1-4, e.m radiation has the same velocity c, and the same electromagnetic nature, but may have different frequencies. The relation between frequency, f, and wavelength, λ, is valid for all types of e.m radiation and is given by

$$\lambda f = c \qquad \text{(Equation 1.1)}$$

Accordingly, as the wavelength decreases, the frequency increases.

Besides its wave characteristics, e.m radiation is also described as having a particle-like character. In some cases, light acts as if it consisted of discrete particle amounts or quanta of energy called photons. Each photon carries a discrete amount of energy E, given by the relation:

$$E = hf = hc / \lambda \qquad \text{(Equation 1.2)}$$

where

f = frequency
h = Planck's constant = 6.6×10^{-27} erg-sec
λ = wavelength
c = velocity of light

This equation indicates that the photon energy increases as the wavelength decreases. In many light-matter interactions, the particulate (quantum) nature of light dominates the wave nature. Because light can only interact when the photon energy hf has a suitable value, in such interactions the wave properties appear to be secondary, such as in diffraction and interference experiments.

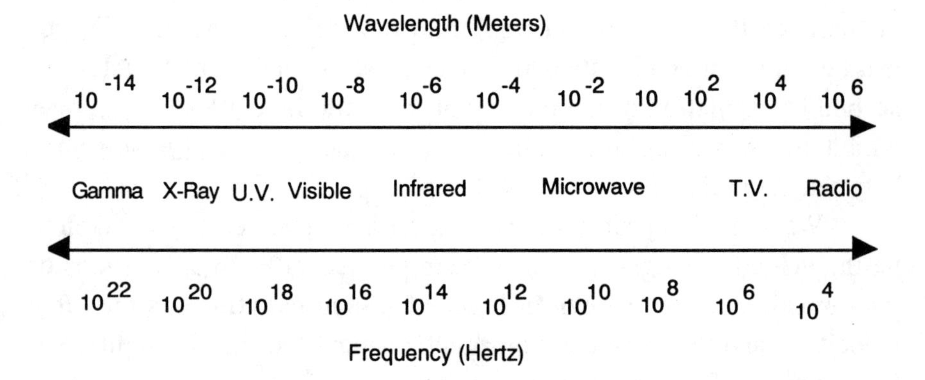

Figure 1-4 The electromagnetic spectrum

1.2.2 Properties of Laser Light

Primary interest in lasers arises from the fact that laser light has properties that are significantly different from that of light from conventional light sources. Laser light is characterized by high degrees of: (i) directivity, (ii) brightness, (iii) coherence, and (iv) monochromaticity. It is these special properties of laser light that allow it to be used for wide practical applications in science and industry. These properties are not independent of each other, but it is convenient to discuss their main aspects separately.

Directivity. Laser light is not a perfectly parallel flux of light; at large distances it gradually broadens due to diffraction. The directivity of the beam is expressed by the angular broadening, Dq, which is related to the beam diameter d, at the exit of the laser and its wavelength, by the relation

$$Dq = \lambda / d \qquad \text{(Equation 1.3)}$$

The small divergence angle of a laser beam allows it to be focused to very small dimensions and therefore to high intensities. The divergence angle is typically expressed in milliradians. The directivity of laser radiation is high because the phase of the light waves over the cross-section of a laser beam is fixed almost everywhere. This uniformity in phase is generally known as coherence. One of the chief characteristics of laser light is that it is coherent in space and time.

Brightness. The brightness (or radiance) of a given source of e.m wave is defined as the power emitted per unit surface area per unit solid angle. Although the brightness of a beam does not change as it propagates, and cannot be changed by any passive optical system, its irradiance (power/area) may be increased by focusing. Because of its very good directivity, laser light can be focused to a diameter equal to only a few times its wavelength using a lens of short focal length. For example, even a small output power of 1 mw focused to an area of 10 mm^2 produces an irradiance of 100 Mwm^{-2}.

Coherence. Coherence is the property of laser light that mainly distinguishes it from other light. A coherent light beam will have three characteristics: (i) the same wavelength, (ii) the same direction, and (iii) the same phase.

The wavelength, as stated before, is the distance between two like points on a wave. The light waves in a laser beam all have the same wavelength—this is also called *monochromatic* light (see below).

The phase of a wave, in its most practical sense, refers to its position relative to another wave. If two waves are in phase, they are lined up in space and time. If the waves are shifted with respect to each other, then they are out of phase by a given amount (see Figure 1-5).

Coherence also causes a phenomenon called laser speckle. Speckle is produced when laser light is scattered from a diffusing surface. Speckle can be used in some measurement applications, but can create problems in others.

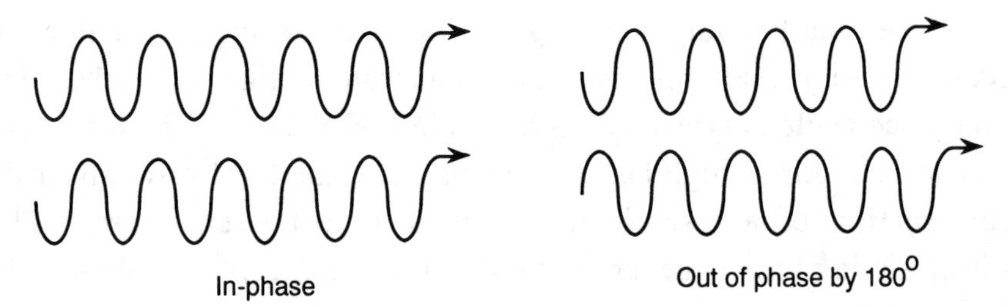

Figure 1-5 Wave phase relationships

Spatial Coherence. Spatial coherence means that the light at the top of the beam is coherent with the light at the bottom of the beam. Spatial coherence describes the phase correlation at two different points across a wave front at a given instant of time. Waves may be spatially coherent but not temporally coherent. The phase relationships in a plane perpendicular to the direction of travel are constant, hence all the waves are in phase in space.

Temporal Coherence (a.k.a. monochromatic). Temporal coherence occurs if two waves in a laser beam remain coherent for a long time as they move past a given point, i.e., they stay in phase for many wavelengths. Each wave has the same constant frequency; therefore, the phase relationships along the direction of travel of the waves are constant.

Monochromaticity. All light sources have a bandwidth greater than zero, including lasers. If a laser could produce exactly one wavelength, laser light would be fully monochromatic. This property of laser light is due to two circumstances: (i) only an e.m wave of frequency, f, given by Equation 1.4 can be amplified, and (ii) oscillation can only occur at the resonant frequency of the resonant cavity. The latter circumstance leads to the laser line width being much narrower than the line width observed in spontaneous emission. Unlike the light waves from ordinary light sources, which are emitted as a succession of irregular pulses, the oscillation of laser light is almost a pure sinusoidal wave over a long period of time.

1.3 Laser Scheme

A laser produces light by combining stimulated emission, a resonant cavity, and a pump source (or excitation mechanism). Figure 1-6 illustrates the scheme for a laser.

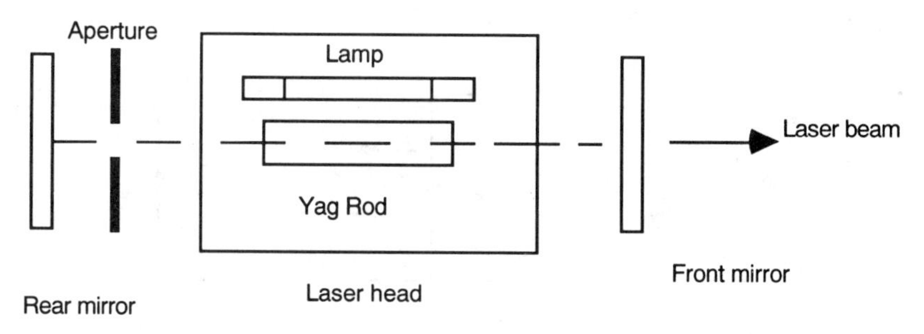

Figure 1-6 Scheme of a laser

1.3.1 Absorption, Stimulated and Spontaneous Emission

A laser exploits three fundamental phenomena that occur when an e.m wave interacts with a material, namely the processes of spontaneous emission, stimulated emission, and absorption. These phenomena, illustrated in Figure 1-7, demonstrate the particulate nature of light. Whenever light is absorbed or emitted by an atomic or molecular system, it always involves a quantum of energy.

Spontaneous Emission. A laser material has an infinite set of energy levels. Assuming that energy level E_1 is less than E_2, where E_1 is the ground level L_1, and the atom (or molecule) is initially in level L_2. If E_2 is greater than E_1, then the atom will tend to decay to level L_1. A corresponding energy difference (E_2 - E_1) must then be released by the atom. When this energy is released in the form of an e.m wave, the process is called spontaneous or radiative emission. The frequency, f, of the radiated wave is given by rearranging Equation 1.2 to give the expression,

$$f = (E_2 - E_1) / h \qquad \text{(Equation 1.4)}$$

where

h = Planck's constant; 6.6×10^{-34} j•s
f = frequency.

Spontaneous emission is therefore characterized by the emission of a photon of energy, $hf = E_2 - E_1$, when the atom decays from level 2 to level 1.

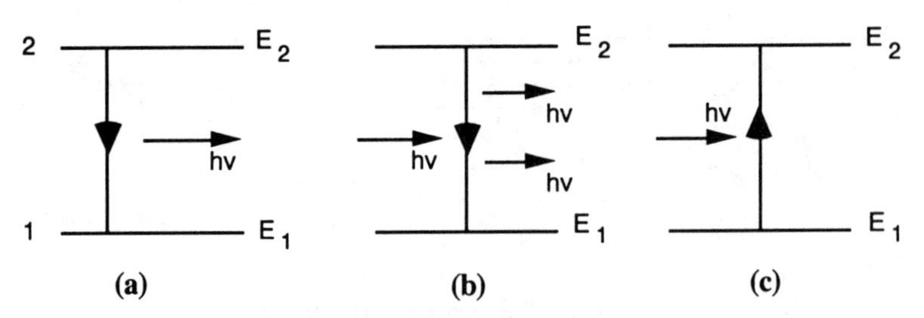

Figure 1-7 Schematic illustration of the three processes: (a) spontaneous emission; (b) stimulated emission; and (c) absorption

Stimulated Emission. If an atom initially exists in level 2, and an e.m wave of frequency $f = (E_2 - E_1) / h$, the same as the spontaneously emitted wave, is incident on the material. Then, since this wave has the same frequency as the atomic frequency, there is a finite probability that this wave will force the atom to undergo the transition from level 2 to level 1. In this case the energy difference $E_2 - E_1$ is delivered in the form of an e.m wave which adds to the incident one; this is called stimulated emission. It should be noted that there is a fundamental distinction between spontaneous and stimulated emission: In the case of spontaneous emission, the atom emits an e.m wave that has no definite phase relationship with the wave emitted by another atom, and the wave may be emitted in any direction. In the case of stimulated emission, since the process is forced by the incident e.m wave, the emission of any atom adds in phase to that of the incoming wave, which also determines the direction of the emitted wave.

Absorption. If the atom is assumed to be in level 1 initially (the ground level), then the atom will remain in this level unless some external stimulus is applied to it. If an e.m wave of frequency f given by Equation 1.4 is incident on the material, there is a finite probability that the atom will be raised to level 2. If the energy difference (E_2 - E_1) required by the atom to undergo the transition is obtained from the energy of the incident e.m wave, then this is the process of absorption.

1.3.2 Population Inversion

There are many types of amplifying medium that can be used in a laser through which light is amplified by population inversion and stimulated emission. In the normal state of a laser medium, there are many more atoms in the lower level than in the upper level. If the medium is excited by an appropriate method so that the number of atoms in the upper level N_u is greater than the number of atoms in the lower level N_l, then the light incident on the medium will be amplified by stimulated emission. This is the process of amplification.

The process of making N_u greater than N_l at thermal equilibrium is *population inversion.* In order to invert the population of an atomic level, the atoms have to be excited by depositing energy in the medium by using a method to decrease N_l atoms in the lower level and increase the number of N_u atoms in the upper level. Since atoms are redistributed as if pumped from the lower level to the upper level, this process is called pumping. Common methods of pumping include optical pumping, where atoms are excited by the illumination of light; excitation by electric discharge, in the case of gases; and by the infusion of carriers with a forward current through a semiconductor junction.

1.3.3 Pumping Schemes

Because absorption predominates over stimulated emission at thermal equilibrium, where level 1 is more populated than level 2, the incoming e.m wave would cause more 1 to 2 than 2 to 1 transitions. But this does not produce population inversion because a condition will be reached where both populations are equal ($N_1 = N_2$), in which case the absorption and stimulation process compensate each other. This is referred to as two-level saturation. It becomes necessary therefore to use more than two levels of the infinite set of levels in an atomic system. Figure 1-8 shows three- and four- level laser pumping schemes that can be used to produce population inversion.

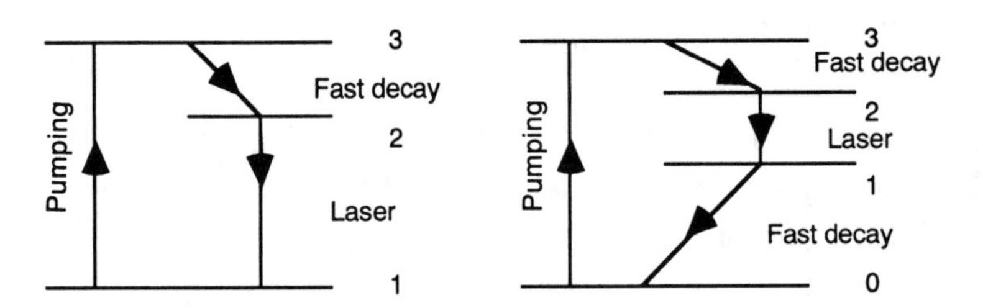

Figure 1-8 (a) Three-level and (b) four-level laser schemes

In a three-level laser scheme, the atoms are pumped from level 1 to level 3. If the material is such that these atoms decay rapidly to level

2, then a population inversion occurs between level 2 and level 1. In a four-level laser scheme, atoms are pumped from the ground level (0) to level 3. If the atoms then decay rapidly to level 2, then population inversion occurs between level 2 and level 1.

1.3.4 Resonant Cavity

The final requirement for a laser is a resonant cavity that comprises a geometrical structure such as two parallel mirrors. To achieve laser action, a resonant cavity is required so that the light will make many passes through the active medium. Such an arrangement allows the light to travel a long distance in the medium (Figure 1-9).

For resonance to occur, an integral number of half wavelengths is needed between the mirrors. Laser action only occurs at discrete wavelengths satisfying the relationship,

$$q = (\lambda / 2) \times d \qquad \text{(Equation 1.5)}$$

for some integer of q, where

d = mirror separation
q = an integer much greater than unity
λ = wavelength.

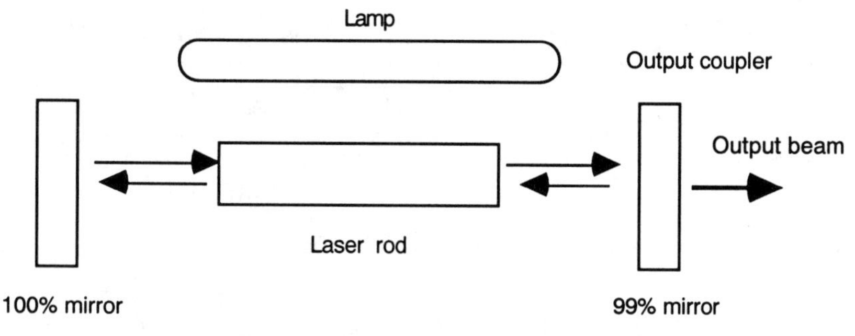

Figure 1-9 Typical resonant cavity

The terms cavity and resonator are used interchangeably in laser technology. All laser cavities share two characteristics that complement each other: (i) they are basically linear devices with one relatively long optical axis, and (ii) the sides parallel to this axis are open rather than closed. Cavities designed to meet these criteria may have different shapes and are not always designed for the lowest energy loss.

A simple resonator is a device that consists of a pair of mirrors which are aligned plane-parallel to each other. One mirror is placed at each end of the laser media, with one mirror a total reflector while the other acts as a partial reflector (or output coupler). This allows part of the of the generated laser beam to pass outside the cavity.

An output coupler allows a portion of the laser light to leave the laser in the form of a beam. The amount of light allowed to escape varies from one laser to another; from less than 1% for some helium-neon lasers to more than 80% for some solid-state lasers.

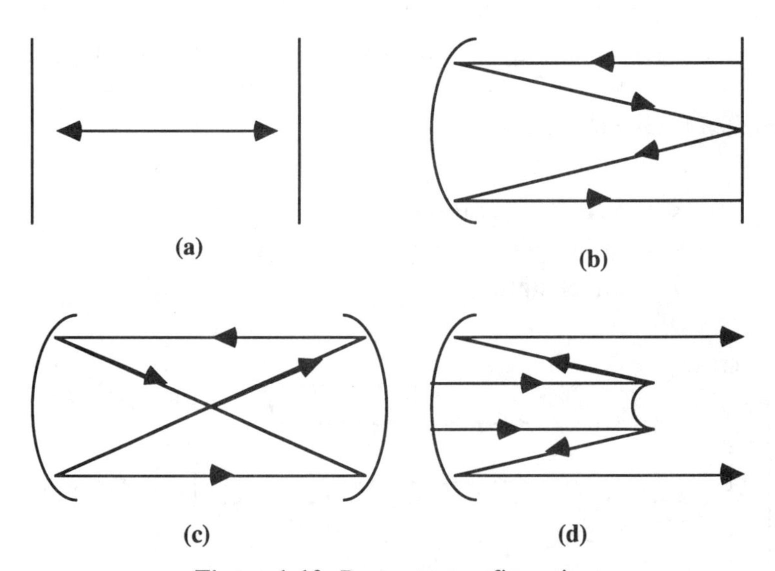

Figure 1-10 Resonator configurations

The oscillation of laser light takes place in the cavity that is defined by the mirrors at each end. Because cavity length is several times longer than the wavelength of the laser beam, it is possible to oscillate on several modes simultaneously. To limit oscillation modes, the laser cavities are opened with only a pair of small mirrors at opposite ends. Several resonator configurations are possible. The simplest is the plane-parallel resonator called the Fabry-Perot resonator (Figure 1-10a). Other configurations include the confocal resonator (b), hemifocal resonator (c), and the confocal unstable resonator (d).

Laser resonators are described as stable or unstable. Stability refers to the condition where the threshold of stability is reached if a light ray initially parallel to the cavity axis could oscillate between the mirrors forever without escaping from between them. Resonators that do not meet the stability criteria are called unstable resonators because light rays diverge away from the axis. But the design of unstable resonators collects higher volumes of laser energy leading to higher overall conversion efficiency than with the stable resonator.

1.3.5 Laser Amplification

If you consider the two arbitrary energy levels in a given laser material, where N_1 and N_2 are their respective populations, it can be shown mathematically that the material behaves as an amplifier if N_2 is greater than N_1, while it acts as an absorber if N_2 is less than N_1 at thermal equilibrium condition. When the material acts as an amplifier, then a population inversion exists in the material. This means that the population difference $N_2 - N_1 > 0$ is opposite in sign to that which exists under normal thermal equilibrium conditions ($N_2 - N_1 < 0$).

1.3.6 Gain

If more atoms are in the upper level of the transition than in the lower level, then there will be more stimulated emission than absorption, and the radiation will be amplified as it propagates. In such a case there is said to be gain at the resonant frequency. The gain of laser photons due to stimulated emission is not only proportional to the number of atoms in the upper level, but also to the number of photons already in the cavity. The efficiency of the stimulated emission process depends on the type of atoms used and on other factors, which are reflected in the size of the amplification or the gain coefficient.

1.3.7 Threshold

In order to sustain laser oscillation, the stimulated amplification must be sufficient to overcome loss effects in the laser cavity. These losses include scattering and absorption of radiation at the mirrors, as well as the output coupling of radiation in the form of the usable laser beam. This sets a lower limit on the gain coefficient, below which laser oscillation does not occur. The condition in which the gain coefficient is greater than or equal to this lower limit is called the threshold condition for laser oscillation.

1.3.8 Summary of Laser Theory

The basic structure of a laser consists of an amplifying medium with inverted population between two mirrors. The two mirrors constitute a resonator that confines light at resonant frequency. Excitation energy is vigorously supplied to the active media to produce the specific condition called population inversion, where more atoms of the laser media are in a specific excited-state energy level than in the lowest (ground) level. An atom in an excited state may release excess energy by spontaneous emission of light in discrete units called photons. The unique feature of a laser device lies in the fact that because of population inversion, the energy release may also be accomplished by the process known as stimulated emission.

In the case of stimulated emission, a photon released by an excited atom will cause an excited atom in its path to release a photon of excess energy. The result of this interaction is the combination of two photons with identical coherence properties (phase relationship), so that they add together to produce a beam of twice the intensity. For the excited laser media, its amplitude rapidly increases while its coherence properties remain unchanged. On reaching the total reflecting mirror, the beam direction is completely reversed, thus allowing another pass through the excited laser media so that the beam may be further amplified. When the beam reaches the partial reflecting mirror, a portion of it escapes. This escaping portion is the active emission from the laser. This process will continue as long as sufficient pump energy is supplied to the laser media.

1.4 Output Characteristics

1.4.1 Output Modes

Laser resonators have two types of modes—transverse and longitudinal. Transverse modes manifest themselves in the cross-sectional profile of the beam (its intensity pattern). Longitudinal modes correspond to different wavelengths within the gain bandwidth of the laser. The lowest order transverse mode, where intensity peaks at the center of the beam, is called TEM_{00} mode (transverse electromagnetic mode, zero-zero order). For many applications, the TEM_{00} single mode produced by stable resonators is considered the best quality beam. But multimode beams deliver more power in a poorer quality beam.

1.4.2 Beam Diameter and Divergence

The light emitted by a laser diverges as it moves through space. Beam divergence angle is usually expressed in milliradians (1 mradian = 0.0573°). Divergence is a measure of the angle at which the beam spreads after leaving the laser, and is usually less than 10 mradians. Beam divergence decreases with increases in output aperture or by using shorter wavelengths. It should also be noted that manufacturers often specify the "half-angle beam divergence" as the divergent angle of the output beam (Figure 1-11). Beam diameter and divergence are determined by the cavity optics and vary depending on the type of laser. CW gas lasers generally have the smallest values of beam divergence (< 1 mradian). Semiconductor lasers emit as much as 30° (0.524 radians) of full-angle divergence.

1.4.3 Beam Focusing

Focusing ability is important in many laser applications. Some lasers are capable of being focused to what is called a "diffraction-limited" beam spot. This is the smallest spot size attainable by any given optical system. It also means a laser beam cannot be focused infinitely smaller. In geometrical optics, it is shown that diameter of the focused beam is approximately equal to the focal length of the lens, multiplied by the angle of divergence. As values of divergence increase, a lens of short focal length will concentrate more power on the focal area.

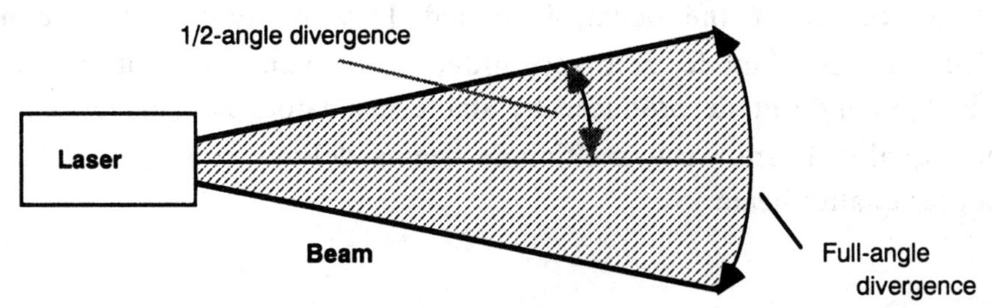

Figure 1-11 Full-angle and 1/2-angle beam divergence

1.4.4 Continuous Wave Beam

A cw laser beam's intensity is measured in terms of power radiated. The beam undergoes little or no fluctuation with time, creating a steady flow of coherent photons. Many gas lasers produce cw output because the gas can be designed to flow through the lasing chamber not only to replenish the gas, but also to act as a cooling device.

CW lasers often require long periods of time (minutes to hours) to stabilize to the beam's intensity for very constant operation. A laser operating with a cw output for a period greater than or equal to 0.25 second is regarded as a cw laser. The irradiance of a cw beam is measured in watts per centimeter squared (or watts per square inch), and is referred to as power density.

1.4.5 Pulsed Beam

A beam with a duration of < 0.25 second is said to be a pulsed beam. Its intensity is measured in terms of joules per centimeter squared, and is called energy density. The term "pulse width" means the duration of the pulse. It is technically defined as the total time required for the pulse to rise from zero intensity, build to a maximum, and then fall to zero again. If the beam is repetitively pulsed, the repetition rate (prr), in pulses per second, is measured in hertz (one pulse per second = 1 Hz).

1.4.6 Ultra-Short Pulses

The laser can generate an output of nearly constant amplitude and phase that may be modulated at very high speeds. Amplitude and frequency modulation up to microwave frequencies can be obtained. Ordinarily, in electronics, the limit on the pulse width or response time is about 1×10^{-9} second (1 ns). Laser pulses may be obtained which are 1000 times shorter (1 ps) or less.

1.5 Modified Laser Outputs

A physical model of a typical laser is not just a closed loop system consisting of two-level atoms and an optical resonator. Rather, the laser is an open system interacting with the external environment. Laser operation can be enhanced by either modifying the laser device itself or by modifying the beam it generates. Modifications to the laser apparatus can be done by the manufacturer or by the user. Factory modifications include substitution of different power supplies, choice of resonator optics, selection of control system, and method of packaging. User modifications involve changes in the laser beam and providing flexibility in terms of wavelength, pulse length, power, etc.

1.5.1 Wavelength Selection and Tuning

Some lasers emit at only one wavelength; others can be tuned to emit at a number of different wavelengths. In some cases, manufacturers can determine wavelength when assembling the cavity optics. In other cases, users can select wavelength either by choosing cavity optics or by adjusting a wavelength selective element placed in the cavity.

Wavelength selection is normally made by a wavelength-dispersive element such as a prism or diffraction grating. The dispersive element is placed between the cavity mirrors or serves as a mirror itself. It spreads out the light spectrum and only reflects a narrow range of wavelengths along the cavity axis where it can oscillate. Light at undesired wavelengths is scattered out of the laser medium.

1.5.2 Nonlinear Wavelength Changes

The output wavelength of a laser beam can be altered using the nonlinear effects and harmonic generation. As the beam passes through a nonlinear crystal, interactions between beam and laser material generate an electromagnetic wave at twice the laser frequency. To obtain peak efficiency, the characteristics of the crystal must be matched precisely to the laser wavelength.

The magnitude of the nonlinear effects is proportional to the square of the laser power. This means high powers are needed to make harmonic generation efficient. Efficiency increases pump power and therefore with the intensity of the fundamental laser beam. Because harmonic generation depends on peak power, not on pulse energy, efficiency can be increased by compressing pulse length, thereby increasing peak power while pulse energy remains the same or is reduced. Harmonic generation is normally used only with lasers that can produce high peak power pulses, such as the Nd:YAG, ruby, and dye lasers.

1.5.3 Raman Shifting

Raman shifting is also a technique that is used for changing wavelengths. When molecules scatter light they may change the photon's energy. If the transition is to a higher energy level, the photon is scattered with a lower energy than it arrived with and therefore has longer wavelength than the incident light (so-called Stokes shift). If the transition is to a lower energy level, the scattered photon carries away the excess energy, and has shorter wavelength and higher energy than the incident light.

Like nonlinear effects, Raman shifting is not likely to occur until high incident power is reached. It can also be used to shift the wavelength of high-power lasers to regions where they are more useful (particularly in downshifting the ultraviolet wavelengths of excimer lasers to longer wavelengths in the visible and near ultraviolet spectrum). This greatly increases the number of wavelengths generated from excimer lasers.

1.5.4 Q-switching

When the lifetime of the upper level of the laser transition is relatively long, a short laser pulse of high instantaneous power can be obtained by a method known as Q-switching. The term Q refers to the so-called "quality factor" of a laser resonator, which measures loss or gain of the cavity. A low Q would refer to a system that would not easily support oscillation; thus to switch from a low Q to a high Q means to change rapidly from a condition in which the laser cannot lase to one in which it will. The mechanics of Q-switching usually incorporate some sort of electro-optical, acousto-optical, or electro-mechanical shutter between the mirrors of the laser cavity.

In the Q-switched mode of operation, the laser is initially pumped continuously while the Q factor of the laser resonator is kept low. One way of doing this is to put a high-loss optical element in the cavity. The high-loss element is suddenly removed when the population inversion has sufficiently increased, and thus the Q value of the resonator is suddenly switched to a high value. As a result, the energy accumulated in the upper level is released as a high-power laser output in a very short time (ns). The peak power output from a Q-switched laser is a large pulse that is considerably higher than that obtained from ordinary pulsed oscillation.

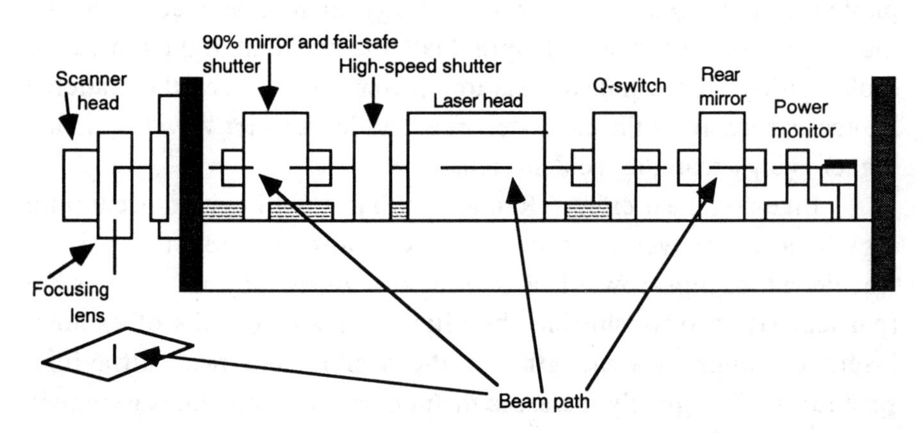

Figure 1-12 Q-switching laser configuration

There are three basic devices used for Q-switching. These are: (i) rotating mirrors or prisms, (ii) active modulators, and (iii) passive modulators. When an optical modulator is used, by blocking off one of the cavity mirrors, it normally does not transmit light. When switched to transparency, the light is able to reach the mirror, so that the cavity Q factor increases to a high level and the laser generates a Q-switched pulse. Modulators are usually electro-optic or acousto-optic devices.

1.5.5 Mode-Locking

The technique of mode-locking allows the generation of laser pulses of ultra-short duration (picoseconds) and very high peak power (gigawatts). Mode-locking refers to the situation where the cavity modes are made to oscillate with comparable amplitudes and with locking phases.

Mode-locking is usually accomplished by inserting an ultra-fast intensity dependent switch, such as a bleachable dye, inside the resonant laser cavity. Since many of these dyes may be "switched" in less than 10^{-13} seconds, it becomes theoretically possible to produce individual laser pulses in this time range. The pulses contained in the pulse train of a mode-locked laser are called picosecond pulses (10^{-12} sec). Mode-locked lasers using saturable dye absorbers are used to produce picosecond pulses with peak powers that may exceed 10^{20} w.

Modulation can be active, by changing the transmission of the modulator; or passive by saturation effects. In both cases interference among the modes produces a series of ultra-short pulses. Mode-locking requires that a laser oscillate in many longitudinal modes, and does not work for many gas lasers with narrow emission lines. The technique can be used with Nd:YAG, dye, and semiconductor lasers. Both pulsed and cw laser operation can be mode-locked.

One mode-locking technique is called the colliding-pulse laser. This is a 3-mirror ring laser with two counter-circulating pulse trains. Pulses in each direction pass through a very thin jet of a saturable dye absorber. The absorption coefficient of the absorber is smallest when the intensity is largest. Therefore the cavity loss is least when the counter-circulating pulses collide and overlap in the thin dye jet. The thinness of the absorber forces the pulses to overlap within a very short distance and hence over a very short time interval ($t = 3 \times 10^{-4}$ sec).

1.5.6 Cavity Dumping

Cavity dumping is basically a technique to couple laser energy directly out of the oscillator cavity without having it pass through the output mirror. In this case, both cavity mirrors are totally reflecting and sustain a high circulating power in the cavity.

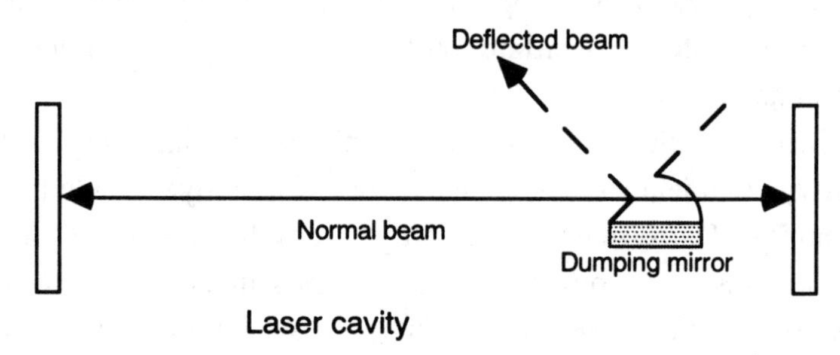

Figure 1-13 Cavity dumping scheme

This circulating power can be dumped out of the cavity by deflecting it. One method is illustrated in Figure 1-13. In this approach, an acousto-optical deflector is put in the cavity. The deflector normally transmits light to the cavity mirrors, but when in the cavity dumping mode, it switches light out of the cavity. Cavity dumping can be used with cw lasers that cannot be Q-switched. It can also be combined with Q-switching and mode-locking to produce special purpose beam characteristics.

1.5.7 Amplification

The output of lasers can be amplified by passing it through a laser amplifier (a.k.a. master oscillator power amplifier, or M.O.P.A.), which is essentially a laser medium without a resonant cavity. In simple cases, the beam makes a single pass through the amplifier where excitation has produced a population inversion. The laser light stimulates emission from the excited species in the amplifier and this increases optical power.

The main purpose of amplifiers is to build up high-energy pulses with high peak power. Pulse energy can be boosted by passing it through one or more amplifier stages. More energy can be extracted from the active medium in this way than when it functions as an oscillator. Oscillator-amplifier configurations are used to extract high-energy pulses from optically pumped solid-state, gas, and dye lasers.

BIBLIOGRAPHY

Cheo, Peter K. (editor). *Handbook of Molecular Lasers.* New York: Marcel Dekker, Inc., 1987.

Elite Laser Engraver—Maintenance and Safety Manual. Orlando: Control Laser Corporation, 1991.

Facts about: Laser Cutting. Norway: AGA Sweden and Institute for Product Development , 1991.

Hecht, Jeff. *The Laser Guidebook.* New York: McGraw-Hill, Inc., 1986.

Hitz, C. Breck. *Understanding Laser Technology.* Tulsa: Penwell Publishing Co., 1985.

How a Laser Works. Orlando: Control Laser Corporation, 1991.

Laser Technology. Waco, TX: Center for Occupational Research and Development, 1985.

Lengyel, Bela. *Lasers.* New York: John Wiley & Sons, Inc., 1971.

Miloni, Peter and Eberly, Joseph. *Lasers.* New York: John Wiley & Sons, Inc., 1988.

Ready, John. *Industrial Application of Lasers.* New York: Academic Press, 1978.

Sasnett, Michael. *Kilowatt-Class CO_2 Lasers Meet Present and Future Industrial Needs.* Palo Alto: Coherent General, 1991.

Schafer, Franz P. *Dye Lasers.* New York: Springer-Verlag Series, 1973.

Shimoda, Koichi. *Introduction to Laser Physics.* Tokyo: Iwanami Shoten Publishers, 1982.

Svelto, Orazio and Hanna, David. *Principles of Lasers*. New York: Plenum Press, 1982.

Thygarajan, K. and Ghatak, A.K. *Lasers—Theory and Applications*. New York: Plenum Press, 1981.

Winburn, D.C. *What Every Engineer Should Know about Lasers*. New York: Marcel Dekker, Inc., 1987.

2

TYPES OF LASERS

Introduction

Among a very large class of hundreds of laser materials, only a few are frequently used in many of the most successful lasers. It is difficult to predict which laser materials will work well, and many became prominent based on their performance after the laser was developed. Future developments in lasers will change the list of materials used and this will lead to the development of new lasers operating at different wavelengths.

Lasers are often classified according to the type of lasing medium used. At present, gas lasers appear to be the most successful and are most widely used in industry. Of these, the two most successful are the helium-neon and the carbon dioxide lasers. Other important lasers include the semiconductor laser, solid-state laser, ruby laser, and dye laser.

The data and characteristics available are generally representative of a whole category of lasers. It should also be noted that some of the data presented, such as those on power and wavelength, are likely to change and be improved upon in the future.

2.1 He-Ne Laser

Helium-Neon (He-Ne) lasers are common neutral gas lasers. They are compact, portable, and easy to use as a source of visible laser light for alignment and laboratory research. He-Ne lasers can be made to operate at many wavelengths, but most are designed to emit visible (red) light at 632.8 nm.

Table 2-1 provides a quick-reference summary of characteristics for the He-Ne laser.

Table 2-1 Summary for Helium-Neon Lasers

Active Medium	Neon Gas
Output Wavelength*	632.8 nm
Power Range	0.1 mw – 100 mw
Pulsed or CW	CW
Excitation	Electrical (500–3,000-v DC)
Polarization	Unpolarized or Linear

* most common wavelength

Figure 2-1 shows the general structure of a commercially available He-Ne laser.

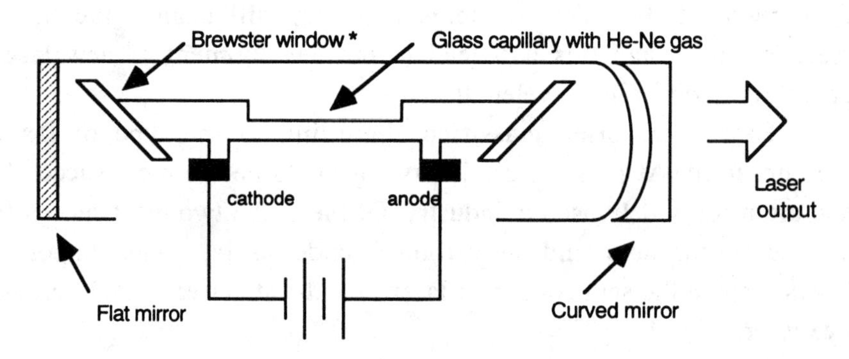

Figure 2-1 Diagram of the He-Ne laser

2.1.1 Principles of Operation

The population inversion mechanism in the He-Ne laser involves a combination of electron impact excitation of helium, and excitation transfer from helium to neon. The gas mixture of helium and neon form the lasing medium, and this mixture is enclosed between a set of mirrors forming a resonant cavity. One of the cavity mirrors is completely reflecting, while the other is partially reflecting, to couple out the laser beam. When a discharge is passed through the gas, electrons are accelerated down the tube where they collide with helium atoms and are excited to higher energy levels.

Figure 2-2 illustrates the relative energy levels of helium and neon. Helium atoms are easily excited to levels F_2 and F_3. These levels are metastable and hence the helium atoms excited to these levels spend a relatively long amount of time before becoming de-excited.

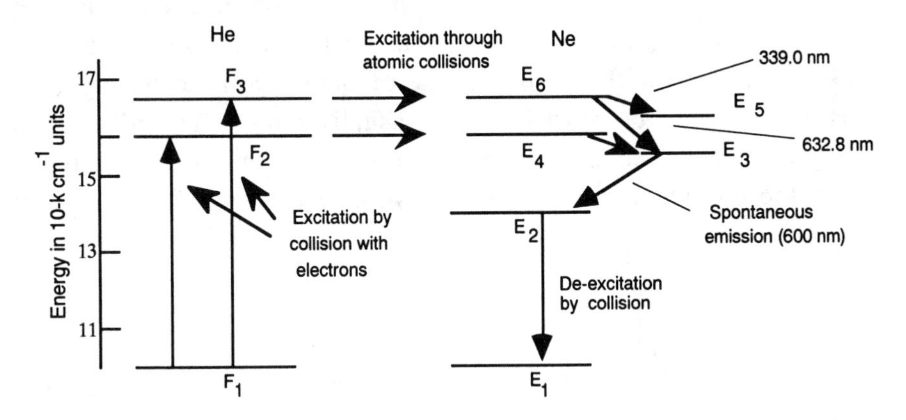

Figure 2-2 (a) Energy level diagram of Helium (b) Energy level diagram of Neon

Some of the excited states of neon correspond approximately with the energy of excited levels of F_2 and F_3 of helium. This means that when the Helium atoms at F_3 and F_2 collide with neon atoms in the ground level E_1, an energy exchange takes place. This results in the excitation of neon atoms to the E_4 or E_6 level. The long lifetime of F_2 and F_3 of helium makes this transfer highly probable. Thus, the discharge through the gas mixture continuously populates the excited energy levels E_4 and E_6 of neon. This helps to create a state of population inversion in neon between the higher levels E_4 and E_6, and the lower energy levels E_5 and E_3.

The various transitions lead to emission by the neon atom at wavelengths of 339 nanometers (nm), and 632.8 nm. Specific frequencies may be obtained by using mirrors which reflect only the frequency required.

The output power as a function of tube current is shown in Figure 2-3. For low tube currents the gas discharge is unstable and there is no output. For currents above a few milliamperes, a stable plasma is produced and the laser output increases with increasing current. At excessively high tube current, the output power saturates and begins to decrease. The addition of a ballast resistor will maintain the tube current within desired limits.

In the He-Ne laser, the gain is the inverse function of the diameter of the gas tube. To maintain population inversion and keep the laser operating, the neon atoms must be able to collide easily in the tube. In order for the collision rate of neon atoms to be high, the diameter of the tube must be small, usually only a few millimeters. The practical consequence of having limits on the diameter is that it limits the output power because the volume of gas cannot be easily increased.

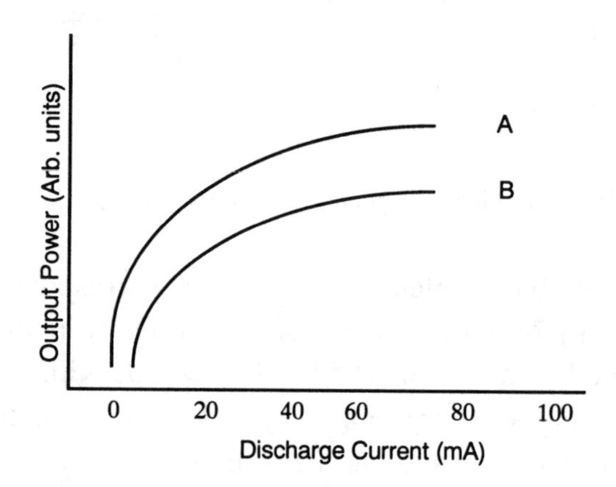

Figure 2-3 Power output as a function of tube current

The pressure in He-Ne laser tube depends on the diameter of the tube, generally a few torrs. The gas mixture is typically 90% helium and 10% neon. The gain of the laser is a function of gas mixture, pressure, tube diameter, and tube current. Commercial lasers are constructed to provide optimum gain for a given set of conditions.

2.1.2 Beam Parameters

Output Modes. He-Ne lasers produce a TEM_{00} beam with gaussian intensity distribution (see Chapter 1 and Chapter 11). The beam generally contains several longitudinal modes unless the laser is specifically designed for single mode operation.

Beam Diameter and Divergence. Beam diameters of He-Ne lasers about 1 mm and tend to increase with power. Divergence is usually about 1 mrad, and drops with increasing beam diameter. Short, low-power models have small diameter beams and large divergences . Long, high-power models may reach a couple of millimeters with about 0.5 mradian divergence.

Power Output. Helium-Neon lasers are available in a range of power outputs from 0.5 mw to 100 mw, in non-frequency stabilized devices. Such lasers typically have amplitude stability of a few percent, which means that the power output varies by a percent over short periods of time. The most common He-Ne laser output powers are 1 mw and 10 mw.

Wavelength. Although it is possible to build a He-Ne laser with other outputs, most operate at 632.8 nm, which is in the red portion of the visible spectrum. A green He-Ne laser, with a wavelength of 543.5 nm, is also becoming widely available.

2.1.3 Electrical and Cooling Requirements

Breakdown Voltage. The voltage-current characteristic of the He-Ne laser tube is also important. There is a region in which the voltage may be high but very little current flows. In order to provide current through the tube, a sufficiently high voltage is needed to "break down" (overcome) the resistance of the gases within the tube; approximately 3,000 v.

After the breakdown voltage is applied, a plasma is created in the tube, which results in a large increase in the current. In order to start the He-Ne laser operating, an initial high-voltage pulse is required, which will momentarily increase the tube's voltage above breakdown. After breakdown, the voltage required to maintain the discharge current is reduced considerably. A typical operating voltage is about 1,350 volts.

Input Power. He-Ne lasers generally require 120 or 240 volts. High peak voltages (about 10 kv) are needed to initiate discharge in the tube.

Cooling. Low-power He-Ne lasers do not produce much waste heat and rely on passive air cooling. High-power models are provided with fan-forced-air cooling.

2.1.4 Common Designs

He-Ne lasers consist of a glass tube that is filled with a mixture of helium and neon gas. The electrodes are mounted inside of the tube which is sealed off. A discharge passes from the cathode to the anode, going through a very small capillary bore (1 mm dia). The capillary structure concentrates the discharge, thus improving overall efficiency. The small diameter of the discharge bore also helps to control the beam diameter, mode, and beam divergence.

He-Ne laser tubes are made with hard seals in which the glass is bonded directly to metal at high temperature. Mirrors are also bonded to the tube, and are not adjustable. Hard seals reduce helium leakage and therefore make contamination from water vapor and other sources insignificant. This extends the life of He-Ne tubes to about 20,000 hours or more.

2.2 Carbon Dioxide Lasers

The CO_2 laser is a very versatile and practical. It produces a output in the far infrared region (over 10,000 nm). A wide range of CO_2 lasers is available, which produce power outputs ranging from low-power (1 w) to high-power lasers (kw class) used in material processing applications.

Table 2-2 Summary for Carbon Dioxide Lasers	
Active Medium	Carbon Dioxide Gas
Output Wavelength*	10,600 nm
Power Range	10 w – 5,000 w
Pulsed or CW	Both
Excitation	Electrical (10,000–50,000 v)
Polarization	Unpolarized

* most common wavelength

Carbon dioxide lasers are available in pulsed or cw outputs. Table 2-2 provides a quick-reference summary for characteristics of the CO_2 laser.

2.2.1 Principles of Operation

Energy Levels. The CO_2 laser is classified as a molecular laser that uses carbon dioxide gas as its active medium. Carbon dioxide has a linear triatomic molecule with three vibrational modes: electronic, vibrational, and rotational.

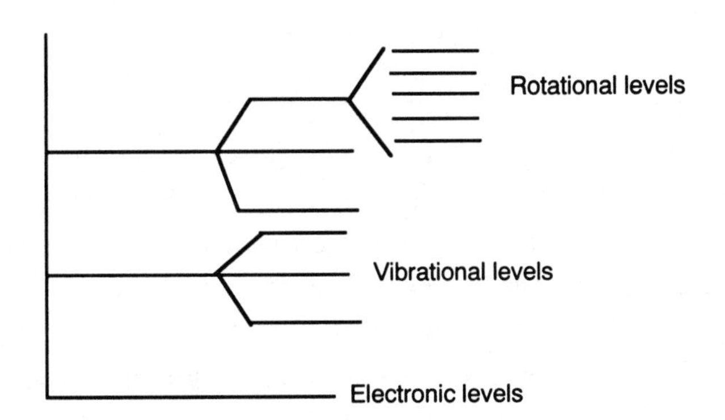

Figure 2-4 Energy levels of a CO_2 molecule

The electronic energy levels are split into vibrational sublevels and each vibrational level is further subdivided into rotational sublevels of motion, as illustrated in Figure 2-4. These vibration modes are shown schematically in Figure 2-5. Energy differences facilitate transitions between the rotational sublevels of a vibrational level and a rotational sublevel of a lower vibration level.

Population inversion in CO_2 lasers is produced through collisions with nitrogen molecules. Nitrogen molecules are excited in the gas discharge by collisions with electrons; they then transfer their energy to the CO_2 molecules. The addition of helium to the mixture may further increase the output power. Helium tends to deplete the population of lower CO_2 levels by collisions and also tends to keep the gas mixture cool because of the high mobility of helium atoms. Practical CO_2 lasers operate with a mixture of CO_2, nitrogen, and helium.

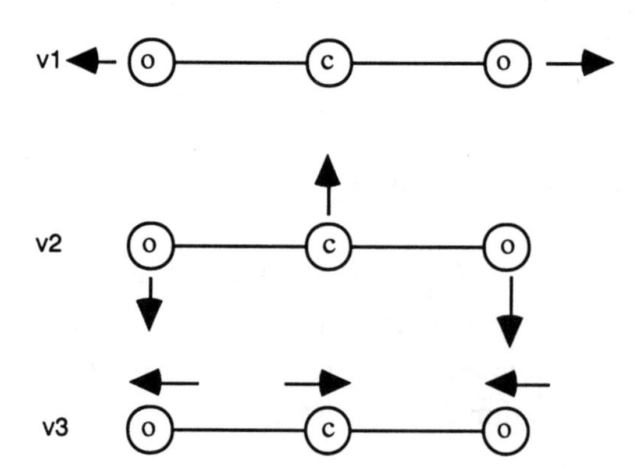

Figure 2-5 Vibrational modes of CO_2

CO_2 lasers are notable for their relatively high efficiency; most are capable of 20–30% efficiency. A majority of the other lasers have low efficiency in converting electrical energy into optical energy. In a typical gas laser, de-excitation from the lower laser level to the ground level involves a sufficient amount of energy which does not contribute to the output of the laser beam. By contrast, in the CO_2 laser, levels involved in the laser transitions are close to the ground level, and hence a large portion of the input energy is converted into the output laser energy.

Cooling Systems. A primary factor that limits the output power of gas lasers is their inability to efficiently remove waste heat from the gas. Air cooling is possible but results in higher temperatures which reduce laser efficiency. Industrial CO_2 lasers usually use recirculating oil and oil-to-water heat exchangers for better system stability and reduced maintenance. Smaller CO_2 lasers may employ water cooling.

An increase of tube current beyond the recommended operating value results in more heat than can be effectively removed from the system in the usual ways employed. Increases in tube diameter also decrease cooling efficiency by increasing the length necessary for helium atoms to reach the walls from the center of the tube. Thus, the most effective method of increasing output power of this type of CO_2 laser is to extend the active length accompanied by an increase in gas flow rate. In much larger systems the gas is recirculated with a few percent being replaced on each cycle.

2.2.2 Beam Parameters

Output Modes. The output modes of a CO_2 depend on the design of the cavity. Often beam quality is sacrificed for higher output powers, although there are some designs that provide both. CO_2 are available with TEM_{00}, but higher power models often make use of an unstable resonator design that produces a different mode output but allows the use of a totally reflective output coupler mirror. Both single and multiple longitudinal mode designs are available.

Beam Diameter and Divergence. The beam diameter and divergence of the beam depends on the output mode of the cavity and subsequently on the design. Lasers that allow TEM_{00} make for smaller diameter beams with lower divergence than multimode designs.

Power Output. The power output of a CO_2 laser is directly proportional to the length of the laser tube, with output powers of up to several hundred watts possible. In conventional flowing gas laser systems operating at low pressure, it is necessary to construct very long lasers in order to generate high power. The high-power output of CO_2 lasers makes them useful for applications such as welding, cutting, and drilling.

Single-line operation is used on low-power CO_2 lasers and on some TEA models, but is not used for high-power operation. Maximum output also depends on the type of laser. Waveguide CO_2 lasers produce low-power cw output (about 50 w). Fast gas transport lasers operate in the kw range, while the TEA produces the highest power.

Wavelength. The emission spectrum of CO_2 lasers is complex, and there are roughly 100 distinct lines. Particular wavelengths can be selected by placing a diffraction grating or tuning element in the laser cavity. Carbon dioxide lasers may also be operated untuned to obtain higher total power on multiple lines. The strongest output wavelength is 10,600 nm.

2.2.3 Electrical and Cooling Requirements

Input Power. CO_2 lasers operate over a wide range of input and output powers. Waveguide lasers draw 2–3 A from a 120 V In some models, the current powers an RF transmitter operating at 20–30 MHz, which applies its energy to the dielectric waveguide structure. Sealed off CO_2 lasers require 6–10 ma DC at 8–20 kv to produce 1–18 w of power.

The fast gas transport (cw) laser requirements range from 120 V to 460 V, 3-phase. TEA lasers have complex power requirements because of the nature of their pulsed operation. Energy from the main pulse typically comes from a storage capacitor that is charged by a DC high-voltage power supply.

Cooling System. Low power CO_2 lasers may use fan-forced-air cooling. High-power models need water, oil or some other coolant often in a sophisticated chiller or heat exchanger.

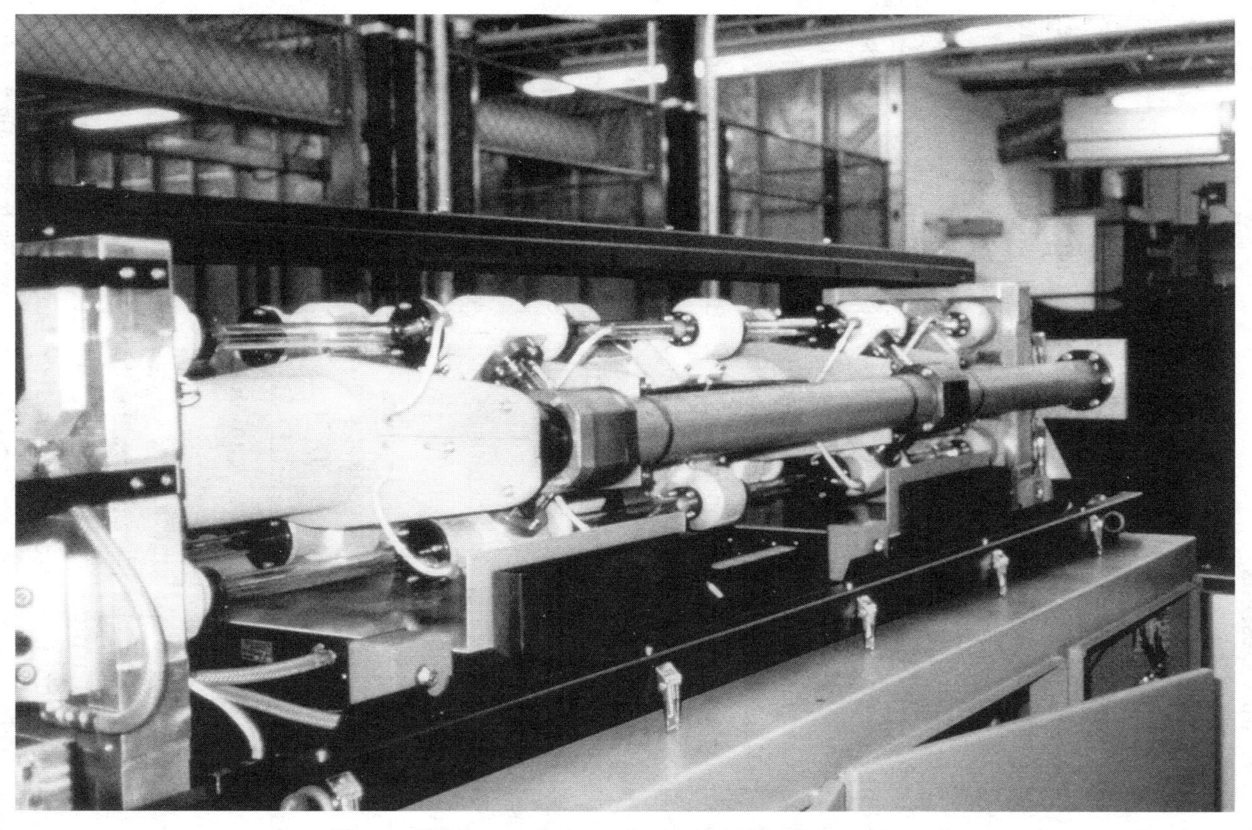

Figure 2-6 Internal view of a typical CO_2 laser system
(*Courtesy of Cincinnati Incorporated*)

2.2.4 Common Designs

The versatility of CO_2 lasers is derived from the several distinct types available; they all have the same active medium but have important differences in internal structure and functional characteristics. Some of the parameters involved include gas pressure, gas flow, types of cavity, and methods of excitation. CO_2 lasers are also classified according to the amount of power they produce.

TEA CO_2 Lasers. Except for the gas dynamic laser, all other CO_2 lasers may be operated in a pulsed mode by applying electrical pulses instead of dc excitation. Pulsed operation is preferred to cw operation for many industrial applications. The wide application of higher-energy pulses of shorter duration led to the development of several types of pulsed CO_2 lasers operating with transverse excitation at atmospheric pressure, referred to as TEA lasers. In TEA lasers, the discharge is transverse rather than parallel to the optical axis. Such an arrangement reduces the electrode spacing to centimeter dimensions. This technique has made it possible to assemble multi-megawatt pulsed gas lasers fairly easily.

The most important characteristic of TEA operation is the use of relatively short discharge paths to excite large volumes of gas at atmospheric pressure. This short, high-volume discharge has two advantages: (i) it makes atmospheric pressure operation possible at easily obtainable voltages (about 20–50 kv), and (ii) it lowers effective resistance of the discharge by several orders of magnitude. This means that a large amount of energy can be introduced for maximizing operating efficiency.

Energy stored per unit volume in the CO_2 gas increases linearly with gas pressure. Thus, greater values for energy per pulse may be achieved at higher pressures. The number of collisions leading to de-excitation of the CO_2 ground level also increases with increased pressure. This provides better gas cooling and means that higher pulse repetition rates are obtainable at higher pressures. As both energy per pulse and maximum power increase linearly with operating pressure, the maximum available average power increases with the square of the pressure. Currently available TEA lasers provide pulse durations in the sub microsecond regime, with total pulse energies ranging from 1 Joule to hundreds of Joules.

Fast-Gas Transport CO_2 Laser. The energy level diagram of the CO_2 laser indicates that a restriction on laser operation occurs in the lower level, which must be depopulated by collisions. Early CO_2 lasers used flowing gas to carry away dissociation products produced by the electrical discharge that had harmful effects on laser operation. If the flow is very fast, the molecules reaching the lower laser level may be swept out and replaced with molecules in the upper laser level which have previously been excited. This will remove the restriction and allow for higher power output, and is the basis for the fast-gas transport laser.

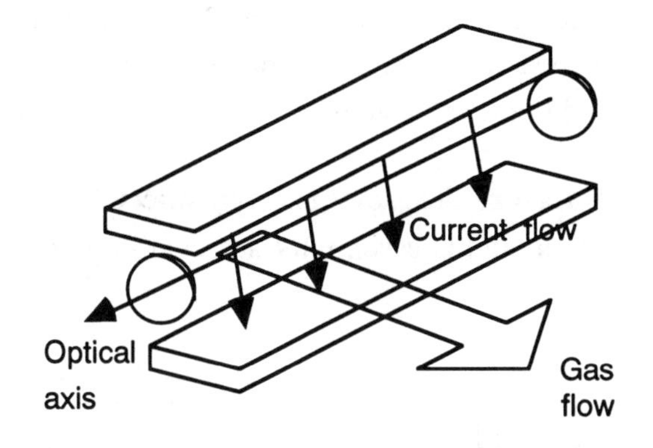

Figure 2-7 Diagram of a Class III cw CO_2 laser

The gas mixture next flows through a quick freeze nozzle (it "freezes in" the excited population inversion) which reduces gas pressure to about 50 torr and increases the velocity to several times the speed of sound. The expansion and reduction in pressure cool the gas very quickly. CO_2 molecules in the upper lasing level remain there, and some molecules in the higher energy states drop to the lasing level. All other energy states are depopulated by the rapid cooling of the gas, and thus inversion is achieved.

The gas travels through the optical cavity at supersonic speed and lasing occurs, dropping CO_2 molecules to the ground state. The gas is exhausted through another set of special diffuser nozzles, which slow the gas further and match its pressure to ambient conditions. The high-power output (kw) produced by such lasers generally require the use of unstable resonators and aerodynamic windows. Other types of molecular gas can also be used in gas dynamic lasers.

The fast-gas transport laser is also referred to as Class III laser. In this laser, gas flow, current flow, and the optical axis are all perpendicular to each other. The illustration in Figure 2-7 is a basic diagram of a Class III cw CO_2 laser.

Typical gas velocities are the same as those of TEA lasers, but the length of the gas flow path is reduced to a fraction of a meter. A typical gas molecule spends only about 2 ms in the active region (about the duration of the lifetime of the upper laser level). Thus, a CO_2 molecule lased from upper level to the ground state is immediately removed from the system. It is then cooled by a heat exchanger and sent through the system again. The optical cavity of the Class III laser is usually folded in order to achieve maximum use of the excited gas.

Gas Dynamic Laser. The cw gas dynamic CO_2 laser requires no electrical excitation, and is essentially a rocket engine with an attached optical cavity.

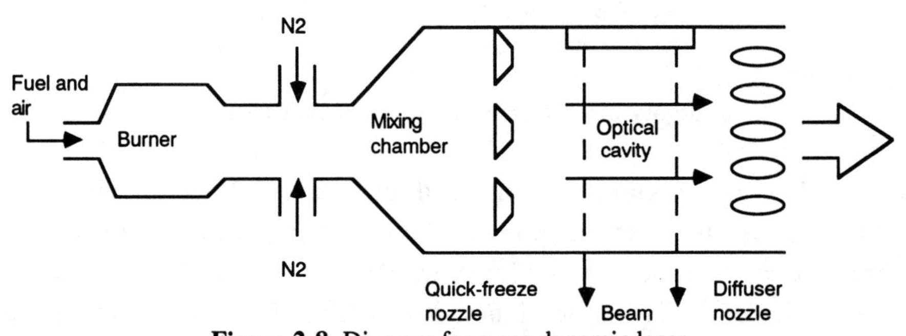

Figure 2-8 Diagram for a gas dynamic laser

The fuel may be cyanogen (C_2N_2), or carbon monoxide (CO), among others. Typically, fuel is burned in a combustion chamber at a temperature of about 1400 degrees Kelvin and a high pressure of greater than 15 atmospheres. The hot gases travel downstream to a mixing chamber, where additional nitrogen is added. Small quantities of water or helium may be introduced at this point. Most of the CO_2 molecules are excited by the N_2 to a high vibrational state (a typical gas ratio is: 90% N_2, 9% CO_2, and 1% H_2O). Figure 2-8 is a diagram of a cw gas dynamic CO_2 laser.

Electron Beam Controlled CO_2 Laser. One of the problems with ordinary discharge lasers occurs because the free electrons in the plasma have two different functions. Electrons must move through the discharge under the influence of the applied electric field, producing new electron-ion pairs by collision to offset losses due to recombination and diffusion to the walls. If the electric field is too low, the electron concentration decreases and the discharge goes out.

The same electrons must excite the gas molecules by collision in order to populate the upper laser level and produce the inversion necessary for laser action. The value of the electron temperature that is needed for optimum laser operation may be different from the value required to maintain a stable discharge. The two functions may be separated by using an externally produced high-energy electron beam fired into the laser region to maintain the discharge.

Such a discharge uses a high-energy (100–200 keV) electron beam to ionize the gas. A field across the gas accelerates the resulting electrons and provides electrical excitation of the laser molecules. The discharge cannot be sustained without the electron beam. The provision of an external ionization agent separates charge production in the discharge from the electric field or transport process. Separation of the source of ionization from the excitation process avoids the problems of self-sustained breakdown and arc formation.

Waveguide CO_2 Lasers. These are small lasers with typical lengths of 5 to 25 cm and bore diameters as small as 1 millimeter. The bores of these laser tubes are made of beryllium oxide. The hollow dielectric structure acts as a waveguide for the CO_2 laser light producing a low-loss optical cavity. The small bore diameter results in good gas cooling efficiency and high gain. Waveguide CO_2 lasers produce output powers of around 0.2 w per cm of tube length. Thus, a laser only 10 cm long can produce an output power of 2 watts. Waveguide CO_2 lasers are rugged and dependable and are attractive for applications in communications, pollution monitoring, and optical ranging systems.

Class II CW CO_2 Laser. In this laser the gas is circulated through the system by a high-speed blower. Gas velocity in the laser tube ranges from 100 to 500 m per second. The primary cooling mechanism is convection, rather than conduction to the walls. The heated gas passes through a water-cooled heat exchanger that removes waste heat. Common characteristics of this type of CO_2 laser are:

- Available output powers of greater than 600 w/m
- Tube diameters of 8–15 cm
- Tube currents of 700 ma

In this type of laser, a single CO_2 molecule is actually in the active region of the tube for less than 0.01 second. The CO_2 molecules are removed from the lasing region, cooled, and introduced into the lasing volume again in the ground state. High efficiencies of the heat exchanger and gas flow system make water cooling of the plasma tube less critical. Figure 2-9 diagrams a Class II CO_2 laser.

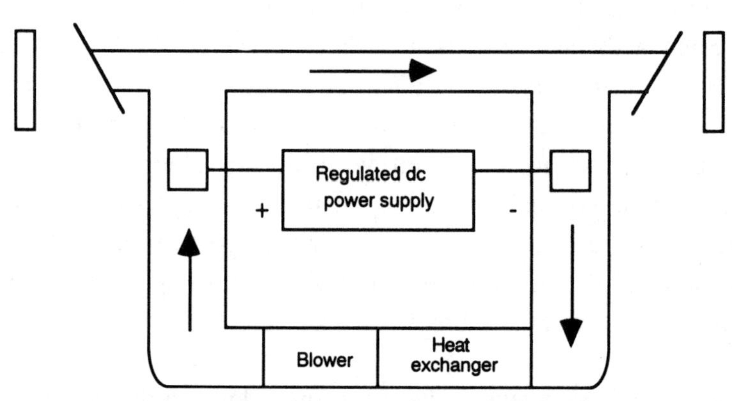

Figure 2-9 Diagram of a Class II CO_2 laser

The efficient removal of waste heat also means that higher tube currents may be used to obtain higher output powers. Because tube walls are no longer involved in the thermal transfer, larger diameters may be used without degrading laser output. Several commercial class systems are available in the 1–8 kw power range. Most are folded systems, and have water cooled mirror mounts and rigid resonator frames. Some also employ the unstable resonator cavity configuration shown in Figure 2-10.

It consists of a concave mirror and a convex mirror arranged to have a common center of curvature. Both mirrors have reflectivity greater than 99%. Light reflects back and forth within the optical cavity, with part of the light passing around the convex mirror to form the output beam. This cavity configuration is usually used only on very high-power systems in which partially transmitting mirrors cannot withstand the high output power flux. The mirrors are constructed of metal and are water cooled.

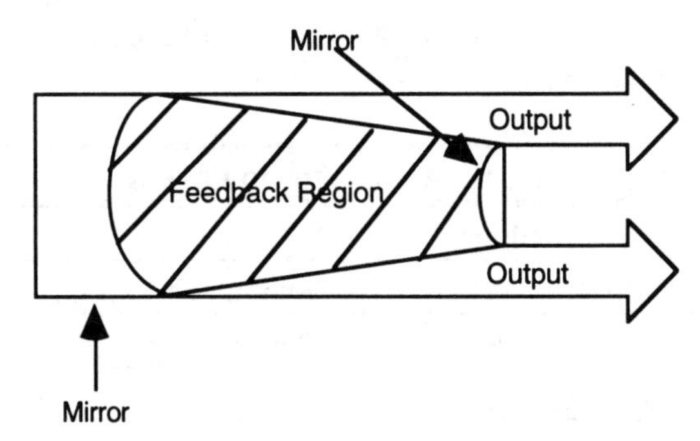

Figure 2-10 Representation of an unstable resonator cavity

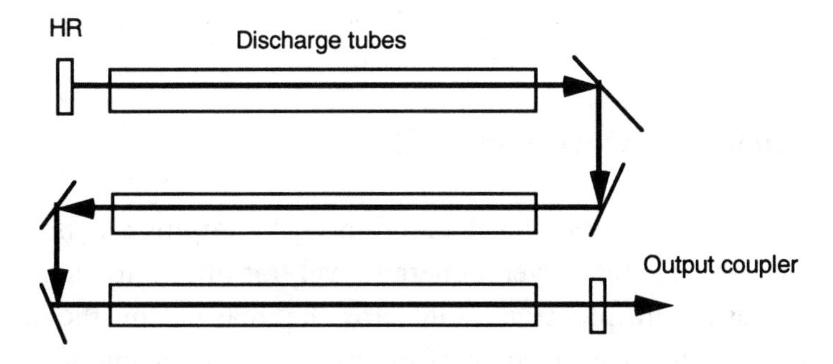

Figure 2-11 Folded resonator (arrows indicate path of beam)

The output power can be increased even more by using a folded resonator design like the one shown in Figure 2-11. This design increases the effective length of the cavity without increasing its actual length. The folded resonator with two or more tubes can produce beams of greater than 1 kw. At these powers, water cooled mirror mounts (and sometimes unstable cavity configurations) are necessary.

2.3 Argon Laser

The active medium of an ion laser is an atomic gas that has been ionized. The argon laser has an active medium of argon atoms with a single electron removed (Ar^{+}). Argon lasers generally emit several wavelengths in the visible spectrum and are used in spectroscopy and as pumping sources for dye lasers.

Table 2-3.1 provides a quick-reference summary for characteristics of the Argon laser.

Table 2-3.1 Summary for Argon Lasers

Active Medium	Argon Gas
Output Wavelength*	488 nm or 514.5 nm
Power Range	10 mw – 10 w
Pulsed or CW	CW
Excitation	Electrical
Polarization	Unpolarized

* most common wavelengths

2.3.1 Principles of Operation

A simplified energy level diagram of the argon ion is shown Figure 2-12. Notice that several energy level transitions are capable of lasing. These multiple transitions are the reason for the laser's multimode operation. Since some of the transitions share energy levels, it is possible that one transition may cancel out another. Each transition has its own probability of occurring so that the multiple wavelengths have various output powers.

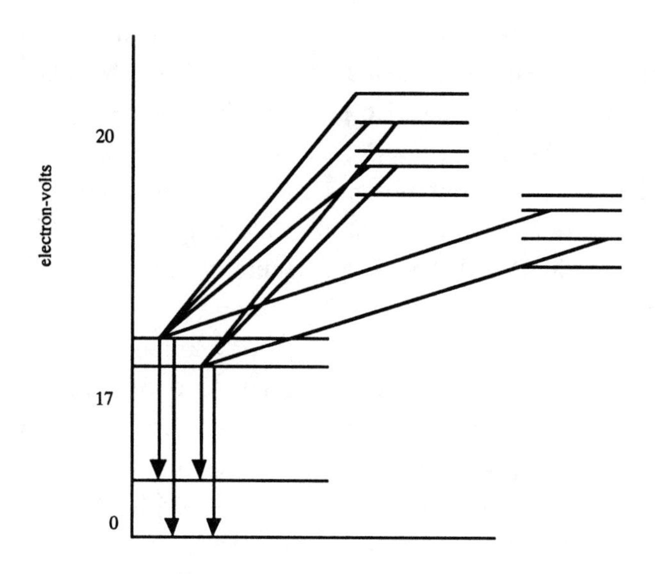

Figure 2-12 Energy level diagram for an argon ion

The argon atom takes 36 eV of energy to ionize. Since each electron collision imparts between 2 and 4 eV, the atom must collide with several electrons before it ionizes (subsequent collisions are necessary to excite the ion after the initial 36 eV). The multiple electron collisions must occur in a short time span, so that the atom does not have time to release its energy in between collisions. A large number of electrons in a small space is necessary for imparting enough energy to the atom to ionize it. This high current density is accomplished by supplying a large amount of current to the laser, confining the tube to a small diameter and applying the magnetic field described below.

2.3.2 Beam Parameters

Output Modes. Argon lasers output a TEM_{00} beam when in single mode operation. Multiple longitudinal mode and single mode operation are available.

Beam Diameter and Divergence. The size and divergence of the argon beam are usually comparable to that of He-Ne and similar gas lasers (0.5 mm diameter and 1.6 mradian divergence).

Power Output. Output powers for the argon range from several milliwatts up to 7 or 8 watts. Multimode outputs have higher powers than single mode. Argon lasers are generally operated with continuous wave outputs.

Wavelength. Argon lasers are capable of lasing at several wavelengths simultaneously (see Table 2-3.2). Output modes range from ultraviolet through the blue-green portion of the spectrum, but the dominant wavelengths are at 488 nm and 514.5 nm. An argon laser that has no tuning mechanism will produce a laser beam that is made up of all the possible wavelengths in a process called *multimode* operation. If a tuning device is installed in the cavity, then it is possible to select one of the wavelengths (usually one of the two dominant wavelengths) for *single mode* operation.

Table 2-3.2 Output wavelengths for the Argon laser.

Wavelength (nm)
514.5
501.7
496.5
488.0
476.5
472.7
465.8
457.9
351.1–363.8

2.3.3 Electrical and Cooling Requirements

Input Power. Most Argon lasers draw high current (10–50 A) and may be operated with 208 volts; or 460 volts, 3-phase.

Cooling. Most argon lasers are water cooled, but some smaller models rely on air cooling.

2.3.4 Common Designs

The basic argon laser is illustrated in Figure 2-13. The power supply has to provide a large current density in order to ionize as well as excite the atoms. The coil around the tube provides a magnetic field that confines the electrons flowing through the tube so they are confined to the center to prevent collision with tube walls. Electrons that collide with the walls of the tube can cause damage and heating. The electrons that are diverted from the tube walls will follow a spiral pattern through the tube, which increases the odds of collision with an atom. Because gas can be lost over time due to atoms embedding in the walls of the tube, the laser is equipped with a gas filling mechanism. The tube is generally mounted in a resonator frame that is designed to maintain the position of the mirrors when the laser expands or contracts during heating or cooling. Water is pumped around the tube to remove excess heat. Since argon lasers are capable of lasing at several wavelengths simultaneously, the cavity may include a tuning mechanism (prism or etalon) for selecting particular wavelengths.

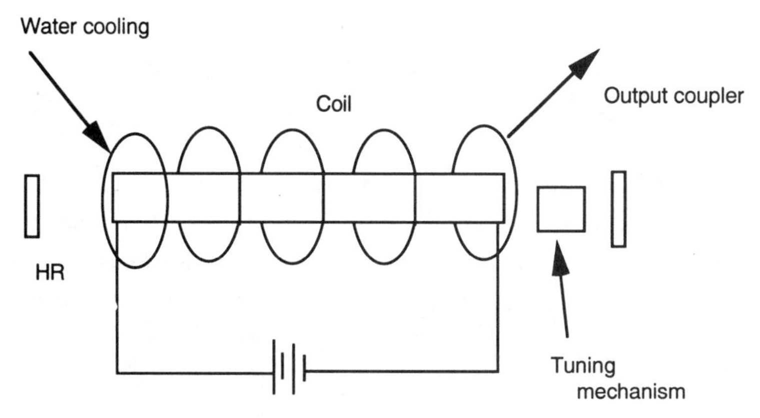

Figure 2-13 Diagram for an argon laser

2.4 Nd:YAG Laser

The most practical solid-state laser is the YAG laser which has a high thermal conductivity, which is ten times that of glass, and emits at a wavelength of 1,064 nm or 1,320 nanometers. YAG is an acronym for yttrium-aluminum-garnet ($Y_3Al_5O_{12}$), a crystalline manmade substance. A typical YAG laser rod is a cylinder 2 inches long, and 5/32 of an inch in diameter. The YAG rod is not pure; it has 2% of a rare earth element called neodymium uniformly distributed throughout the YAG. A neodymium-doped YAG is referred to as the Nd:YAG.

Table 2-4 provides a quick-reference summary for characteristics of the Neodymium:Yttrium-Aluminum-Garnet laser.

Table 2-4 Summary for Nd:YAG Lasers

Active Medium	YAG-doped Nd crystal
Output Wavelength*	1,064 nm
Power Range	10 w – 4,000 w
Pulsed or CW	Both
Excitation	Optical (Krypton lamp)
Polarization	Unpolarized or linear

* most common wavelength

2.4.1 Principles of Operation

Figure 2-13 shows the energy-level diagram of an Nd:YAG laser. Lasing is dependent on the rapid transitions from the lower lasing level to the ground state by radiationless transitions. These transitions occur at a high rate only if the rod temperature is low. Thus, lasing efficiency depends mainly on cooling efficiency. Lower operating temperature could result in higher output powers. Cooling systems are generally operated at temperatures just above the threshold of this effect.

Nd:YAG crystals are excited by absorbing light from a Krypton flash lamp. The crystal absorbs energy in two 730–760 nm and 790–820 nm pumping bands. Krypton lamps provide light in both bands, and cause the molecules in the crystal to excite to the E4 pump band shown in Figure 2-14. The molecules radiate heat in the $E_4 \rightarrow E_3$ transition and the $E_2 \rightarrow E_1$ transition. This heat has to be removed by cooling the crystal rod.

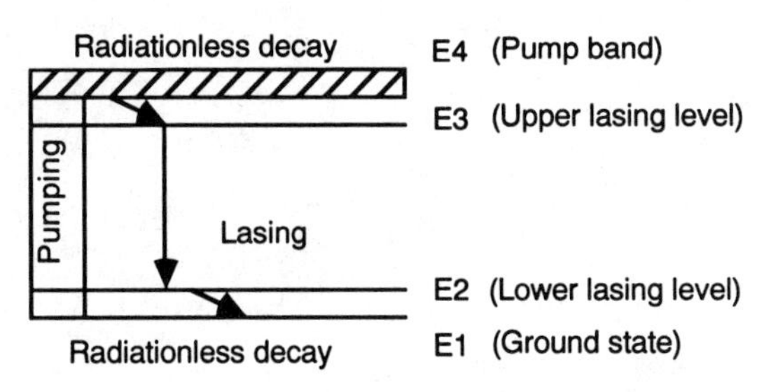

Figure 2-14 Nd:YAG energy-level system

2.4.2 Beam Parameters

Output Modes. Multimode output provides higher powers while single-mode output has better beam quality. Unstable resonators offer a combination of high power and good beam quality, plus efficient extraction of energy from the laser rod.

Beam Diameter and Divergence. Beam diameters are generally 1–10 mm; larger diameters are possible with beam expanders. Divergence ranges from fractions of a milliradian to about 10 mradians.

Output Power. Output power may range from 0.1w to a few kilowatts in some models. When Q-switched at about 10 to 20 ns, an Nd:YAG laser can produce peak powers of hundreds of kilowatts.

Wavelength. The Nd:YAG laser exhibits significant gain at wavelengths between 1,052 and 1,338 nm, but its wavelength is quoted at 1,064 nm. Harmonic generators can be used to multiply the frequency by 2 to 4 times, thus dividing the wavelength by the same factor.

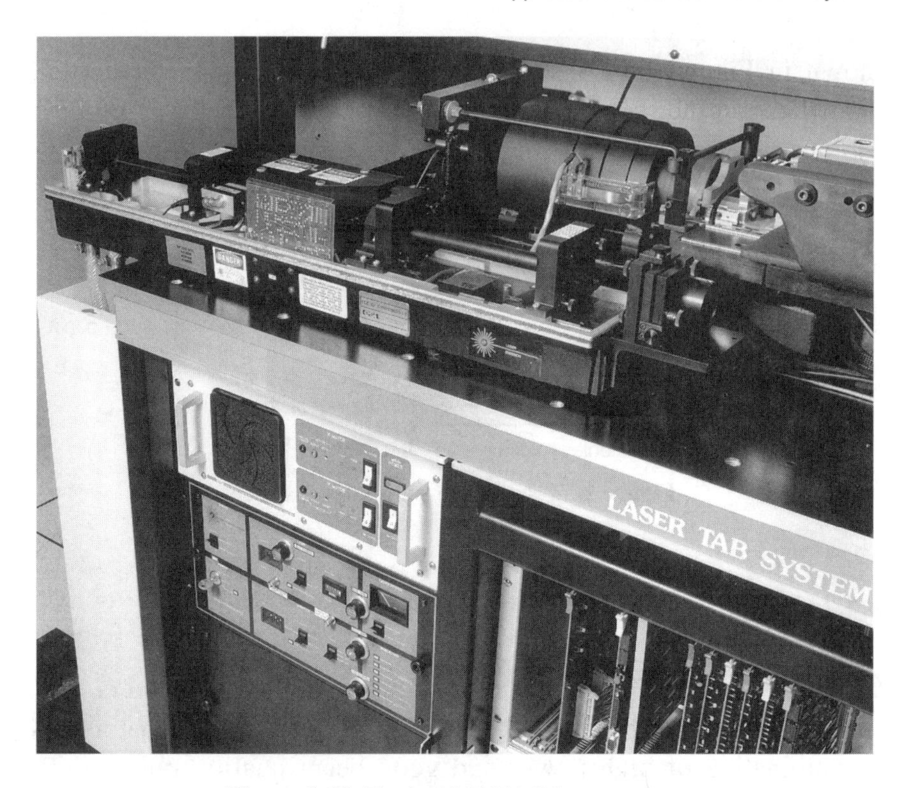

Figure 2-15 Typical Nd:YAG laser system
(Courtesy of Electro Scientific Industries, Inc.)

2.4.3 Electrical and Cooling Requirements

Input Power. Low power YAG lasers may be operated from 24 to 28-v batteries, or they may draw about 500 w from 115-volt AC outlets. Larger models draw tens of kilowatts from 3-phase, 240-v supplies.

Cooling System. Low-power YAG lasers may rely on conductive or air cooling. Industrial class YAG's use open cycle water cooling. Small models may use closed-loop water cooling as an option.

2.4.4 Common Designs

YAG Laser Cavity. The YAG laser rod is placed in a gold-plated elliptical cross-section laser head. Inside the laser head is an elliptical space with the rod at one foci of the ellipse and a krypton lamp at the other foci. All of the light emitted by the lamp is focused on the rod, as illustrated in Figure 2-16. Other geometries, such as the star-shaped head, are used to accommodate lamps.

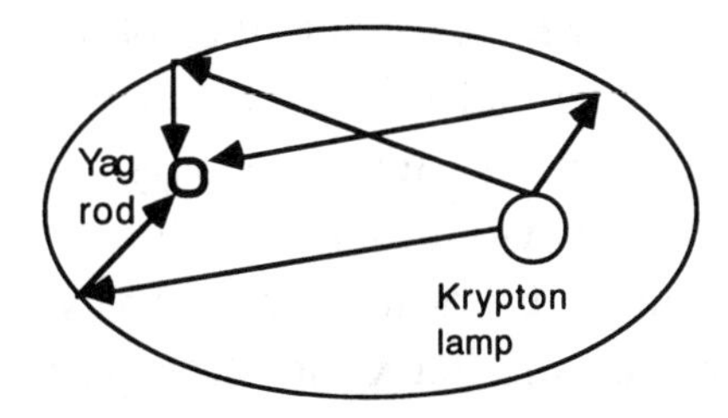

Figure 2-16 End view of a YAG laser cavity

Laser Material. The laser material is shaped into a cylindrical rod whose ends are ground and polished to be plane parallel. When the rod is placed between two mirrors facing each other, and is strongly irradiated by an intense light source around it, a pulse of light is emitted.

The rods used for cw operation are usually from 1–4 mm in diameter and are from 1–6 inches long. Smaller diameter rods are preferred because they present fewer cooling problems than larger rods. The rod ends are usually anti-reflection coated for the Nd:YAG wavelength of 1,064 nm.

The rod is mounted inside a quartz or glass water jacket. Cooling is provided by water flow directly across the rod surface. The rod ends are held in place and sealed by O-rings recessed in the ends of the rod holders to protect them from the pump lamp light.

Optical Pumping System. YAG lasers are usually pumped by optical excitation. The optical pumping for cw Nd:YAG lasers may be a quartz-halogen lamp or a krypton-arc lamp. If a quartz-halogen lamp is used, cooling is applied to the lamp ends. Krypton-arc lamps are generally enclosed in their own water jackets and have water cooling from the lamp cathode. The lamps are commonly mounted with the rod inside an elliptical pumping cavity, which is usually water cooled. New designs have incorporated banks of laser diodes for excitation. Diodes provide the advantages of being air cooled, and having lower power consumption.

Optical Cavity. The optical cavity of the Nd:YAG laser usually consists of two mirrors mounted separately from the laser rod. Several cavity configurations may be used, but all employ at least one spherical mirror. Both long radius and long radius hemispherical cavities are commonly used. In some systems, shaping of the beam cavity is desirable and two mirrors with different radii of curvature are utilized. The hemispherical radius mirror has a reflectivity of about 99.9% and the output coupler transmission varies from less than 1% on small lasers to about 8% on larger ones. The optical cavities of Nd:YAG lasers are often equipped with adjustable or interchangeable apertures for selection of multimode or TEM_{00} operation.

Cooling System. The cooling system is one of the most critical subsystems in a laser. Small lasers may use open-loop cooling systems with water flowing across the rod. Larger systems use closed-loop cooling with water or a water-glycol solution. The coolant is usually refrigerated, but a water-to-water or water-to-air heat exchanger may also be employed.

The cooling fluid circuit begins with the laser rod for maximum rod cooling. The water then flows across the lamps and the laser cavity. A flow switch is generally included to turn the lamp power off if the water flow is interrupted. Loss of cooling will quickly destroy seals, lamps, and the laser rod itself.

2.5 Ruby Laser

Ruby was the material used when laser operation was first demonstrated in 1960. Ruby is sapphire called crystalline aluminum oxide (Al_2O_3) in which a small percentage of aluminum has been replaced by chromium (about 0.05%). The thermal properties of ruby vary greatly with temperature. Ruby absorbs light in the green and blue portions of the light spectrum and emits red radiation at a wavelength of 694.3 nm. The emission has a spectrum approximately 0.4 nm wide at room temperature. Table 2-5 provides a quick-reference summary for characteristics of the Ruby laser.

Table 2-5 Summary for Ruby Lasers	
Active Medium	Chromium-doped sapphire
Output Wavelength*	694.3 nm
Power Range	1–100 joules
Pulsed or CW	Pulsed
Excitation	Optical (Xenon lamp)
Polarization	Linear

* most common wavelength

2.5.1 Principles of Operation

The optical quality of the ruby is a critical factor in its operation. Not only are easily detectable scattering centers detrimental, but so are all variations of the optical path from one end to another. The mode structure and pattern of the radiation generated by ruby lasers are largely determined by optical path variations. Defects in the ruby crystal and errors in its preparation result in an increase of the threshold energy required and in the deterioration of the far field radiation pattern. An energy level diagram of ruby is illustrated in Figure 2-17.

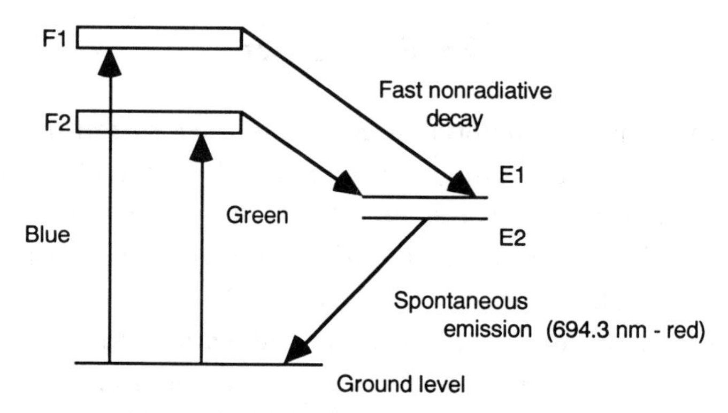

Figure 2-17 Ruby energy level diagram

The Ruby Rod. The dimensions of the ruby rod are determined by the ability to grow crystals of good quality. It is difficult to obtain ruby rods of good optical quality that are longer than 6 inches in length. The diameter is also limited by the necessity for having the pump lamp uniformly irradiate the entire volume of the ruby. This sets practical limits on the diameter of ruby rods to between 0.5–1 inch.

Internal Structure. Solid-state lasers including ruby have two kinds of cavity—the pump cavity and the resonant cavity. Because of the very high pumping energy required, efficient output coupling, as well as reflection in the resonator, are crucial in ruby lasers. Temperature control is also important and in many cases the cooling water flows through the coupling cavity.

Ruby operates well in an oscillator-amplifier configuration in which a pulse from a ruby oscillator passes through a second ruby rod that amplifies it. Commercial ruby lasers may incorporate up to four amplifier stages, which is one of the best ways to produce high energy pulses with good beam quality.

Excitation Mechanism. In the ruby laser, only a small fraction of the electrical input of the exciting lamp is converted into useful energy. Because much of this radiation does not reach the ruby, a practical ruby laser requires at least 100 J of electrical input per cubic centimeter of ruby to operate. The time during which the excitation energy is delivered is also important because the excitation in ruby at room temperature decays with a time constant of 3 milliseconds. Since the energy and power levels are large, the optical pump system must be designed so the heat developed in the system can be removed fast enough to prevent an intolerable rise in temperature for all the components.

Optical pumping of ruby is possible by means of blue and green light because of the presence of two absorption bands in ruby. Xenon-filled photographic flash lamps, when properly operated, emit a significant fraction of their optical output in the desired spectral region. These flash lamps are used either in the form of helical coils surrounding the ruby crystal, or in the form of straight rods placed alongside the ruby rod or in the focal line of a reflector.

A typical pumping circuit (Figure 2-18) used for the operation of a flashlamp has a resistor in the order of 1000 ohms, an inductor, and a capacitor selected to conform with the specifications of the tube.

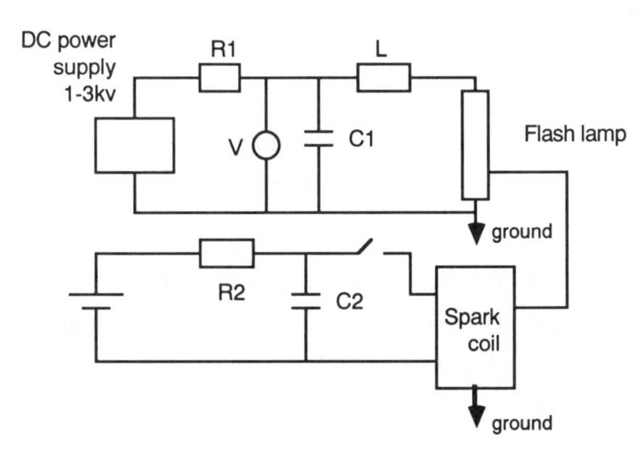

Figure 2-18 Schematic of an optical pumping circuit

The initiation of the discharge through the flashlamp requires a voltage of 10 to 15 kv. The voltage is produced by obtaining a spark from a spark coil connected to a wire wound around the flashlamp. The tube may also be fired by coupling the spark in series with the tube, using a transformer.

The manufacturers of flashlamps provide limiting parameters, usually in the form of curves or formulae specifying the maximum energy dissipation in the tubes as a function of flash duration. The circuit must be designed so that a pulse with a given energy cannot be of less duration than the tube data specify.

Output Characteristics. There is no output from a ruby laser until the pump power has reached a minimum value, called the threshold. Typical threshold values for ruby lasers, which use linear flash lamps that are close-coupled to the ruby, are usually a few hundred joules. Above the threshold, the output is an increasing function of input. Typical values for efficiency are a few tenths of 1%. The limiting factor on output appears to be how much energy can be discharged into the flash lamps without damage. Cooling a ruby laser below room temperature can increase the output energy by up to 50%. The reflectivity of the output mirror also affects output.

2.5.2 Beam Parameters

Output Modes. Ruby lasers can be designed to produce a single longitudinal mode or multimode outputs depending on what is required for the application. Transverse modes are usually the gaussian, TEM_{00}.

Beam Diameter, and Divergence. Beam diameter ranges from 1–25 mm, with divergence ranging from 0.25–7 mradian. Lasers used for holography typically have beams close to the diffraction limit, but some multimode models have large divergence and beam diameter.

Power Output. The peak power radiated from a laser without pulse intensity control is not definite since peaks of intensity are not regular. The output energy of typical ruby lasers often ranges from 1–10 Joules (in normal pulsed lasers). For Q-switched ruby lasers, output powers in excess of 10^9 watts are possible. However, above a few hundred megawatts the ruby may be damaged by high optical fluxes.

Wavelength. Oscillator-amplifier configurations can produce pulses with energy well over 100 J. Average power is limited by low repetition rates.

2.5.3 Electrical and Cooling Requirements

Input Power. Ruby lasers typically operate from single–phase 120-v AC or 240-v AC supply. Initially, peak line current of 10–20 A is drawn to charge a capacitor bank which discharges the high voltage (5–10 kv) through the flash lamp.

Cooling. Typical designs circulate deionized water through the laser head and a heat exchanger that transfers excess heat to air or flowing tap water.

2.6 Semiconductor Lasers

The development of semiconductor diode laser technology has been accelerated by the use of fiber-optics in communications, and by the need for compact, light, and inexpensive sources of optical energy in information handling applications.

Table 2-6 Summary for Semiconductor Lasers	
Active Medium	pn junction of semiconductor
Output Wavelength	visible (red) through infrared
Power Range	0.1 w – 1 w
Pulsed or CW	Both
Excitation	Electrical (5 v)
Polarization	Unpolarized or linear

The distinctive feature of the semiconductor laser is that it lases with a current through a p-n junction and uses very little power compared to other lasers. Semiconductor lasers employ structures and properties that are much different from gas or solid-state. Table 2-6 provides a quick-reference summary for characteristics of the Semiconductor laser.

2.6.1 Principles of Operation

There are two categories of semiconductor diode laser: (i) diode lasers made from compounds which emit in the near-infrared, and (ii) diode lasers made from "lead salt" compounds which emit at longer infrared wavelengths (2,300–30,000 nm). Diode lasers employ a small chip of semiconducting material as the active medium. The most common type of material used is gallium arsenide.

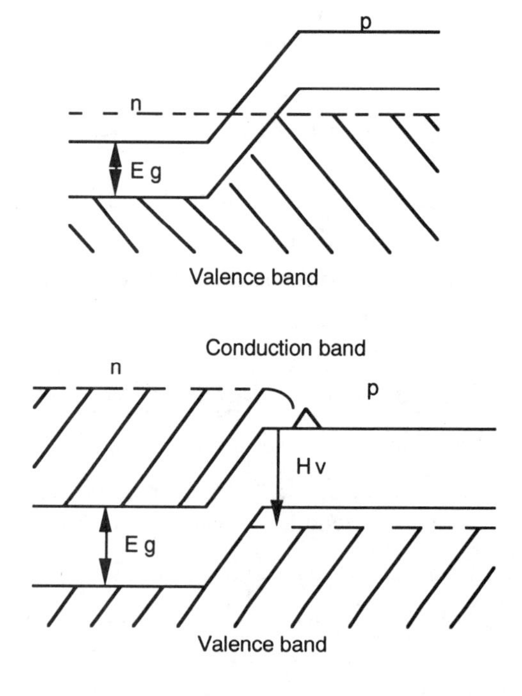

Figure 2-19 Energy levels of semiconductor laser material

In the semiconductor laser, the energy levels involved in the laser action are characteristic of the entire crystalline lattice. These states are not discrete energy states, but are merged into energy bands; i.e., groups of energy states close enough to be regarded as continuous. An energy band diagram of a p-n junction is shown in Figure 2-19. The two important bands are the valence band and the conduction band. The valence band is the highest band filled with electrons. The conduction band lies higher and is separated by a region of energy (the energy gap) in which there are no allowed electronic states.

In order for laser operation to occur, the population must be great enough so that optical gain exceeds optical loss. Thus, the current density through the junction must exceed some minimum value and therefore provide enough holes and electrons so that the radiation generated by their recombination exceeds the losses.

2.6.2 Beam Parameters

Output Modes. Single mode diodes provide narrow linewidth emission, which may be important in applications requiring linear response to modulation. Gain-guided lasers generally produce broad, non-gaussian transverse modes while index-guide lasers produce gaussian, TEM_{00} beams.

Power Output. Most commercially available diode lasers provide a few milliwatts of continuous output. It is possible to obtain more power by using an arrays of diodes or by cooling the diode to very low temperatures. The intensity of the emitted light as a function of injection current is shown in Figure 2-20.

It shows that the intensity increases rapidly above a certain threshold current I_{th}, while below I_{th} it is weak. The threshold current is the starting current for laser oscillation. When the current is below threshold, the directivity of the emitted light is poor and the spectral linewidth is broad; above threshold, laser light has narrow spectral width and sharper directivity.

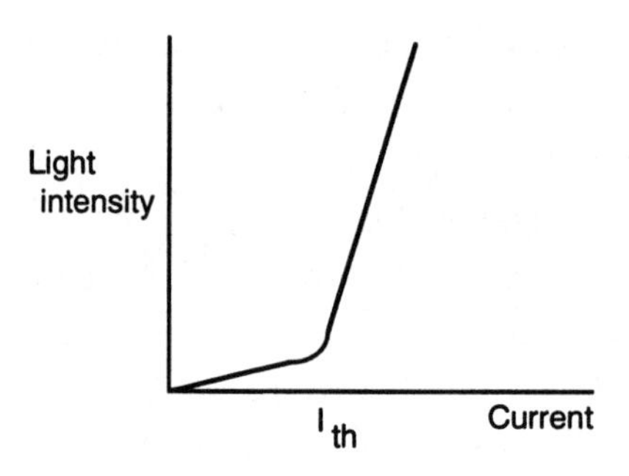

Figure 2-20 Light intensity as a function of current

Beam Diameter and Divergence. Divergence varies with operating conditions, and decreases with output power. Beam divergence is larger for multimode oscillation of gain-guided double heterojunction lasers.

Wavelength. The wavelength of a diode laser is determined primarily by the bandgap of the material in which the holes and electrons recombine. There is an inherent margin of error when fabricating 3- or 4-element diode laser compounds and therefore a wide range of wavelengths are possible with these lasers. Hence, diode laser specifications give a nominal center wavelength of + or - 20–30 nm rather than a precise one. The wavelength of the GaAs laser is approximately 840 nm. Its value depends on several variables, mainly the concentration of impurities, temperature, and current through the diode. Stimulated emission is produced only in a very thin layer about 2 micrometers thick.

2.6.3 Electrical and Cooling Requirements

Input Power. Diode lasers are small and do not require much input power. Most diodes require 2-5 V with a current that depends on laser threshold usually 10–100 mA. The extremely low power required by diode lasers is one of its main attractions for information-handling applications.

Cooling. Most diode lasers are designed for room temperature operation. They usually come with heat sinking devices to remove excess heat. Active cooling with devices such as thermoelectric coolers are used for high-performance applications (see Chapter 11).

2.6.4 Common Designs

Diode Laser Construction. The material for a semiconductor laser is often formed by cleaving the ends of the crystal to form the flat parallel faces needed for an optical cavity. The original material from which the laser is formed is an ingot containing a junction between p-type material and n-type material. Electrical contacts are applied to the top and bottom faces. A heat sink is needed to remove the heat from the laser crystal.

The structure of a simple gallium-arsenide (GaAs) semiconductor laser is shown in Figure 2-21. The two parallel facets of a direct-transition semiconductor are perpendicular to the plane of the p-n junction, where a positive potential is applied to the electrode on the p-type semiconductor and a negative to the n-type. Typical dimensions of a GaAs laser are 1–2 mm with the light emitting region, the junction, only a few micrometers thick. Usually the mirrors for feedback and output coupling are the cleaved ends of the laser diode, without any further coating.

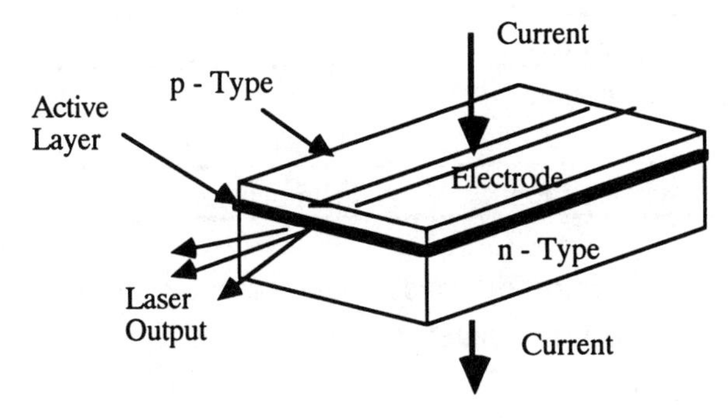

Figure 2-21 Block-construction diagram for a simple diode laser

The reflectivity at the interface between gallium arsenide and air is approximately 36%. Its reflectivity may be increased by coating with metallic films if higher reflectivity is needed to lower the threshold for laser operation.

Excitation Mechanism. Pulse generators capable of providing narrow, high-current, pulsed outputs may be used as the excitation mechanism for injection lasers. Electron beam pumping may also be used.

2.7 Organic Dye Lasers

The organic dye laser is widely used in scientific research because of its unusual flexibility; it promises to provide sources of coherent light easily tunable over considerable bands of the visible spectrum. Dye lasers are also capable of achieving high gain and normally operate at room temperature.

Table 2-7 provides a quick-reference summary for characteristics of the Dye laser.

Table 2-7 Summary for Dye Lasers

Active Medium	Organic dye
Output Wavelength	Wide range
Power Range	mw range
Pulsed or CW	Pulsed
Excitation	Optical (lamp or solid laser)
Polarization	Unpolarized or linear

The versatility of dye lasers also creates complexity in their design. In order to tune wavelengths across a wide range, dye lasers require several changes of the dye solution. The dye degrades and must be dissolved in a solvent, which requires a complex liquid-handling system, and complex optics are needed to produce ultra-narrow linewidth output or ultra short pulses.

2.7.1 Principles of Operation

Active Medium. The active medium of organic dye lasers is an organic fluorescent material dissolved in a common solvent. Typical materials are rhodamines dissolved in alcohol and fluorescein dissolved in water. These substances derive their colors from strong absorption bands in the visible region.

Pumping Mechanism. Dye lasers are excited by optical pumping, using solid lasers in giant-pulse operation or flash lamps that deliver a short pulse with a fast rise time.

Internal Structure. Dye lasers all have the same active medium, but the differences in internal structure are based on application and choice of pumping mechanism. The type of pump mechanism used dictates much of the design of a dye laser because of the energy-transfer kinetics of the dye. The short lifetime (μs) of the upper lasing level makes the pulsed dye laser a high-gain, high-loss system, while the high pump energy needed to pass threshold in cw operation makes it a low-loss, low-gain system.

Spectral Output. The output of dye lasers is a short pulse of broad spectral content. The spectral distribution depends on the solvent used, the concentration of the dye, and other parameters. Because of this dependence, the spectral output is variable and only rough wavelength data can be provided.

2.7.2 Beam Parameters

Output Modes. Like most other characteristics of dye lasers, beam modes are affected by the type of pump source, and optical cavity of the laser. Generally, beam quality tends to be best with cw ion laser pumping, and worse with flash lamp pumping.

CW dye lasers typically produce TEM_{00} output mode beams. Grating tuning or use of intra-cavity components at Brewster's angle produces linearly polarized output. Intra and extra-cavity polarizers can be added to increase the degree of polarization.

Wavelength. Wavelength depends on the particular combination of dye and pump source. Wavelengths ranging from ultraviolet through visible and into infrared are available.

Output Power. Dye laser power is proportional to pump power above threshold. Output power depends on how well the excitation wavelength matches the absorption band of the dye, which makes selection of the pump source vital.

2.7.3 Electrical and Cooling Requirements

Input Power. Laser pumping will use less power than flashlamp pumping. However, power is needed for optical and electrical controls, dye-solution pumps, etc., drawing up to 5 A at 120 v. Flash-lamp pumped lasers use about 15 A from a 120-v source to power the flashlamp.

Cooling System. Typical flash-lamp pumped dye lasers remove excess heat by flowing water through the system to cool both the dye and the flash lamp. In laser-pumped systems, cooling liquid cools the dye solution and flows through the dye cell to avoid degradation of power output.

BIBLIOGRAPHY

Cheo, Peter K. (editor). *Handbook of Molecular Lasers.* New York: Marcel Dekker, Inc., 1987.

Elite Laser Engraver—Maintenance and Safety Manual. Orlando: Control Laser Corporation, 1991.

Facts about: Laser Cutting. Norway: AGA Sweden and Institute for Product Development , 1991.

Hecht, Jeff. *The Laser Guidebook.* New York: McGraw-Hill, Inc., 1986.

Hitz, C. Breck. *Understanding Laser Technology.* Tulsa: Penwell Books, 1985.

How a Laser Works. Orlando: Control Laser Corporation, 1991.

Laser Technology. Waco, TX: Center for Occupational Research and Development, 1985.

Laser Technology For Effective Parts Making. Cincinnati: Cincinnati Incorporated, 1991.

Lengyel, Bela. *Lasers.* New York: Wiley–Interscience, 1971.

Miloni, Peter W. and Eberly, Joseph H. *Lasers.* New York: John Wiley & Sons, Inc., 1988.

Ready, John F. *Industrial Applications of Lasers.* New York: Academic Press, 1978.

Sasnett, Michael. *Kilowatt-Class CO_2 Lasers Meet Present and Future Industrial Needs.* Palo Alto: Coherent General, 1991.

Schafer, Franz P. *Dye Lasers.* Berlin; New York: Springer-Verlag, 1977.

Shimoda, Koichi. *Introduction to Laser Physics.* Tokyo: Iwanami Shoten Publishers, 1982.

Svelto, Orazio and Hanna, David C. *Principles of Lasers*. New York: Plenum Press, 1982.

Thygarajan, K. and Ghatak, A.K. *Lasers—Theory and Applications*. New York: Plenum Press, 1981.

Winburn, D.C. *What Every Engineer Should Know about Lasers*. New York: Marcel Dekker, Inc., 1987.

3 FUNDAMENTALS OF OPTICS

Introduction

Optical components are an essential part of any laser system. An introduction to fundamental concepts in optics will therefore serve as a basis toward the understanding of laser technology. Some of the basic functions performed by optical elements include refraction, reflection, wavelength selection, and polarization effects. Some optical components are known as "passive" because they do not require special control or input power. Others are called "active" because they require some form of control and input power.

3.1 Geometrical Optics

The wave-particle duality of light is a term which refers to the fact that under certain circumstances light behaves as waves, exhibiting typical wave phenomena such as diffraction and interference effects. Under other circumstances, light is said to behave as particles with straight line propagation and particle-like dynamics. Geometrical optics is based on the particle nature of light and deals with light rays and propagation. Physical optics is based on the wave properties of light and includes theories on diffraction and interference. Specific electro-optical systems are described in terms of both theories of optics.

3.1.1 Fundamental Laws

Geometrical optics deals specifically with light as a ray. Fundamental geometrical optics is based on three laws — the law of rectilinear propagation, the law of reflection, and the law of refraction.

The Law of Rectilinear Propagation. The law of rectilinear propagation states that in a uniform homogeneous medium the propagation of an optical disturbance is in straight lines. In other words, unless it passes to a different medium, light travels in a straight line. This line can be represented as a ray.

The Law of Reflection. The law of reflection states that for specular reflection, the angle of incidence is equal to the angle of reflection. This is illustrated in Figure 3-1a. The reflected rays lie in the same plane as the incident ray and the normal to the surface. This plane is referred to as plane of incidence. Most surfaces cause reflected light to contain a portion of specular as well as diffusely reflected light.

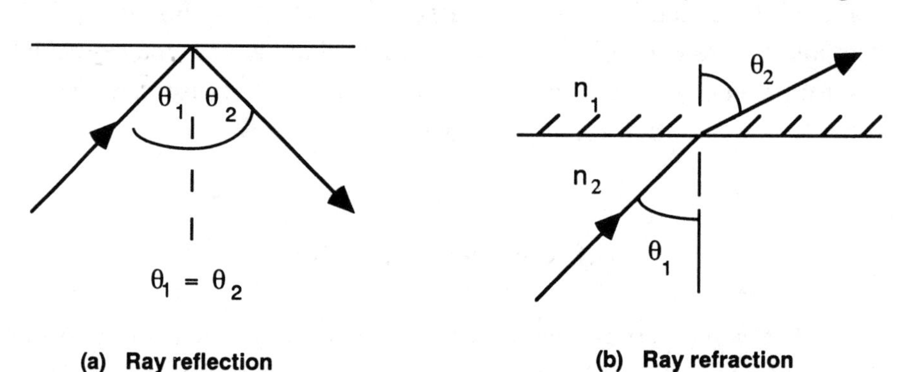

Figure 3-1 Ray diagrams illustrating the laws of reflection and refraction

The Law of Refraction. According to the law of refractive index, when a light ray passes at an oblique angle from a medium of a lesser to a greater optical density (refractive index), it will bend toward the normal. Conversely, a ray passing from a medium of greater refractive index to one of lesser refractive index is bent away from the normal (see Figure 3-1b). This law is also known as Snell's law, and may be expressed by the equation:

$$n_1 \sin \theta_1 = n_2 \sin \theta_2 \qquad \text{(Equation 3.1)}$$

where

θ_1 = angle of incidence
θ_2 = refracted angle, and
n = refractive index of each respective medium.

3.1.2 Reflection and Refraction

Total Internal Reflection. An important phenomenon that relates to Snell's law is *total internal reflection* (TIR). This occurs when light travels from a region of higher refractive index, n_1, into one with the lower of the two refractive indices, n_2.

At an angle of incidence called the critical angle, θ_c, the light reflects rather than refracts. This is known as total internal reflection.

Refractive Index. Refractive index is a measure of the speed at which light travels through a material. The speed of light, c, in a vacuum is used as a reference or standard,* for which the index of refraction is defined to be equal to l. For all other materials, the index of refraction n_{matl}, is calculated as the ratio $n_{matl} = c_{vacuum} / c_{matl}$ and is always greater than 1. Refractive index depends on the nature of the material and the wavelength of the light passing through it. Generally, it tends to increase with material density. As light enters a material at an acute angle, the wave front is bent by an amount proportional to the differences in the wavelength of light in the two materials.

The refractive index of air is small enough so that in practice the refractive indexes of solids are measured relative to air rather than to a vacuum. This not only simplifies the task of measurement, but also

---

* (in a vacuum $c = 3 \times 10^8$ m/second)

gives a more useful value because virtually all optical systems are used in air.

3.1.3 Lenses

Common lenses have surfaces that are shaped like the surface of a sphere or like the section of a cylinder. Spherical lenses focus light in two dimensions; bringing a circular beam down to a point. Cylindrical lenses focus in one dimension; bringing a circular beam down to a line.

Lenses are also classified as positive or negative. Positive lenses bend light rays so they converge, negative lenses bend light rays so they diverge. The focusing power of a lens is normally measured as its focal length. For positive lenses, focal length is approximately taken as the distance from the lens to the focal point where rays initially parallel to the axis come to a point (the ray diagram shown in Figure 3-2a is for a two-dimensional spherical converging lens).

For a negative lens, the focal point is taken as the point behind the lens from which rays appear to diverge. Figure 3-2b shows how an incident plane wave is bent by the lens so that the wave surfaces are diverging from a point in front of the lens.

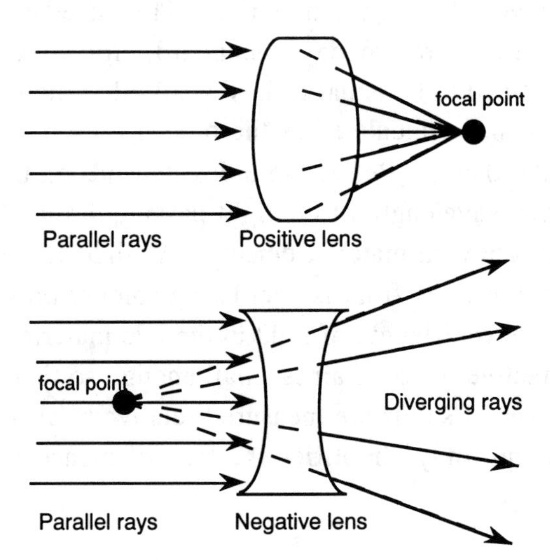

Figure 3-2a Positive (converging) lens **Figure 3-2b** Negative (diverging) lens

As illustrated in Figure 3-3, converging lenses are thicker in the middle than on the edges. They bend the wave front of an incident optical signal, with the middle retarding the wave more than the edge. An incident plane wave will emerge so that the wave surfaces converge to a point behind the lens.

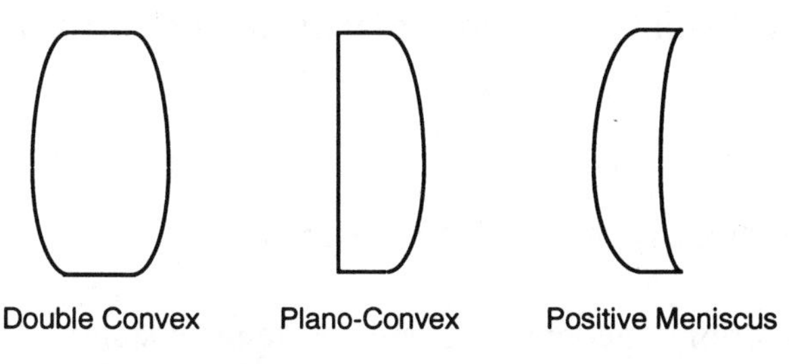

Figure 3-3 Positive (converging) lenses

Diverging lenses are thicker at the edges — see Figure 3-4. (A positive-meniscus lens is thicker in the middle, while a negative-meniscus lens is thinner in the middle.)

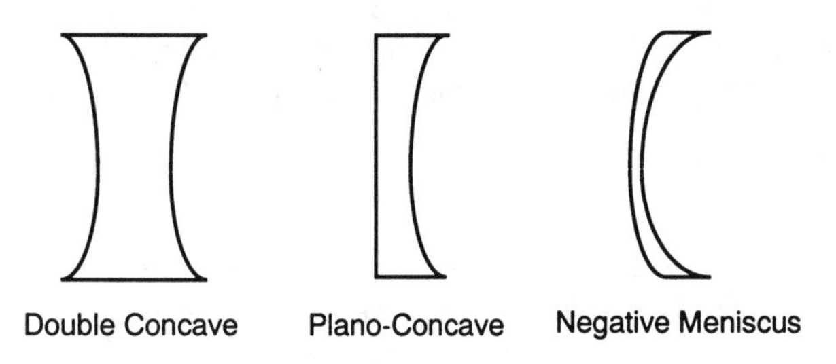

Figure 3-4 Negative (diverging) lenses

3.1.4 Focal Length

Focal length is the distance from the center of the lens to the focal point. It depends on the curvature of the lens and on the refractive index of the lens material. Focal length is used in simple calculations to determine optical characteristics. It is also used to calculate the *focal ratio* F_X, where x is the focal ratio value. Focal ratio is defined as the ratio of focal length to diameter of the lens. Low focal ratio means a short focal length and a working point close to the lens; longer focal ratio means longer focal length and greater working distance.

The focal length that usually appears in optical equations is the effective focal length. This refers to the distance from the optical plane to the principal plane of the lens. The back focal length is the distance from the focal point to the closest intersection of the lens surface with the optical axis.

3.1.5 Nomenclature and Conventions

In describing geometrical optic systems, a standard nomenclature is used. Closely associated with this is a set of conventions that are used in diagramming the system and calculating its values. Common terms are defined below, along with drawing and calculating conventions.

Standard Nomenclature (optic):

Principal axis: The axis running through the geometric center of the lens surface and perpendicular to the surface of the vertex.

Principal focus: A point to which rays parallel to the principal axis converge, or diverge after refraction.

Real image: An image formed by actual rays of light.

Virtual image: An image that only appears to the eye to be formed by light rays.

Focal length: The distance from the vertex to the principal focus.

Center of curvature: The center of the spherical section.

Aperture: A measure of the physical size of the spherical section in a direction lateral to the optical axis.

Conventions (graphical):

- Light initially travels from left to right (except for reflections).
- Rays are drawn so they change directions at an imaginary line drawn through the center of the lens.
- Measurements are made along the optic axis, from the center of the lens.

Conventions (algebraic):

- A positive lens's focal length is positive.
- A negative lens's focal length is negative.
- Real image distances are positive.
- Imaginary image distances are negative.

3.1.6 Sample Geometrical Optics Calculations

Locating Images. The position of an image formed by a lens can be determined by the thin lens equation:

$$1/f = 1/S_1 + 1/S_2 \qquad \text{(Equation 3.2)}$$

where

f = focal length
S_1 = distance from object to lens, and
S_2 = distance from image to lens.

Estimating the Focal Length of a Positive Lens. The focal length of a positive lens can be "roughly measured" by focusing the light from a distant (several meters) source with lens, and measuring the distance from the image to the lens. A simple method for lenses with focal lengths that are few centimeters, is to image an overhead light on to the floor of the lab. Adjust the distance from the lens to the floor until the image is clear. This floor-to-lens distance is roughly equal to the focal length.

Example 3.1

Problem: Locate the image formed by a positive lens (f = 10.0 cm) for an object 25 cm away.

Solution: The image distance is found by modifying Equation 3.2 to solve for S_2; substituting values into the modified Equation; and calculating the answer.

$$S_2 = 1 / (1/f - 1/S_1)$$

$$= 1 / (1/10 \text{ cm} - 1/25 \text{ cm})$$

$$= 16.7 \text{ cm from the lens.}$$

3.2 Physical Optics

The field of physical optics (or wave optics) deals with treating light as an electromagnetic wave. The principles derived from this wave picture are used in the practical applications of lasers and in designing certain optical components. The primary areas of concern in physical optics are diffraction, polarization, and interference.

3.2.1 Diffraction

Because of the wave nature of light, diffraction effects play a major role in the propagation and focusing of laser light. Diffraction is the result of the ability of light waves to interfere with one another and produce constructive and destructive interference patterns. *Diffraction occurs when a beam of light is obstructed or limited in size by an object or an aperture in its path.* Diffracted light will always spread into areas that were not exposed before the aperture or obstacle. Figure 3-5 illustrates the diffraction of light as it passes through an aperture.

Notice that the light waves spread out as they pass through the aperture. This diffraction effect is present in optical systems involving lenses and mirrors whose edges limit the width of the light passing through them. It is diffraction that contributes to the divergence of a laser beam as it passes through the output coupler.

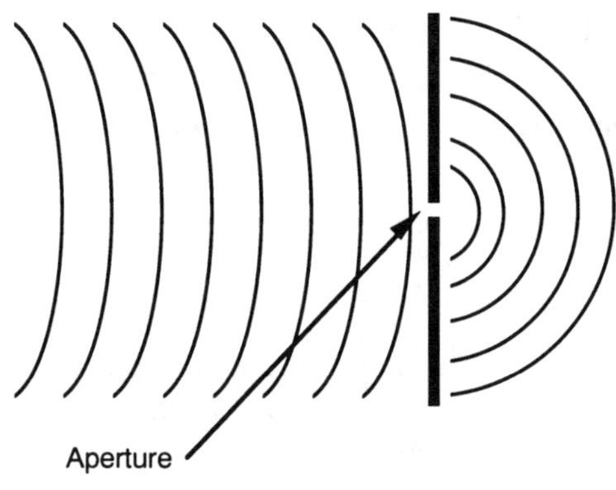

Figure 3-5 Diffraction of light waves passing through an aperture

Diffraction principles are also used to produce an optical component known as a diffraction grating. This component has thousands of apertures (or slits) that intensify the diffraction effect and cause collimated light (such as a laser beam) to split into several rays (or orders). Since diffraction is also a function of wavelength, a grating can be used to split incoming light with multiple wavelengths into separate parts, each with a single (or near single) wavelength and traveling in a separate direction.

3.2.2 Polarization

The electric field in a light wave may have different orientations with respect to the direction of propagation. As light moves through a medium, its electric field is always perpendicular to the direction it travels, but may be oriented several ways. Light that is linearly polarized will always be oriented the same way (see Figure 3-6a). Unpolarized light has a random orientation of the electric field that changes as the light propagates. Some light may be elliptically polarized so that field orientation rotates around the direction of propagation in a set pattern.

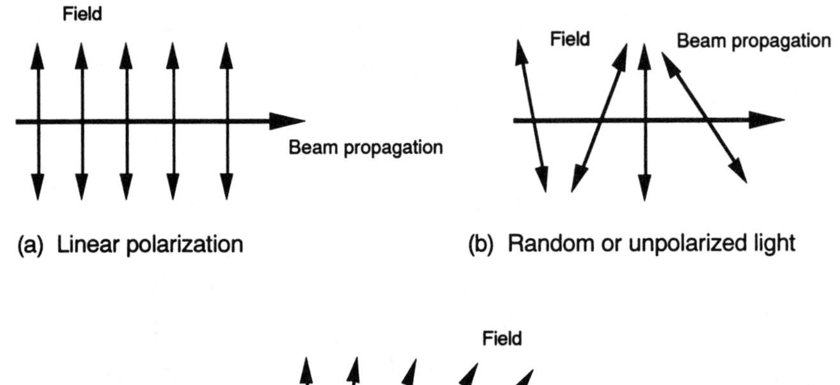

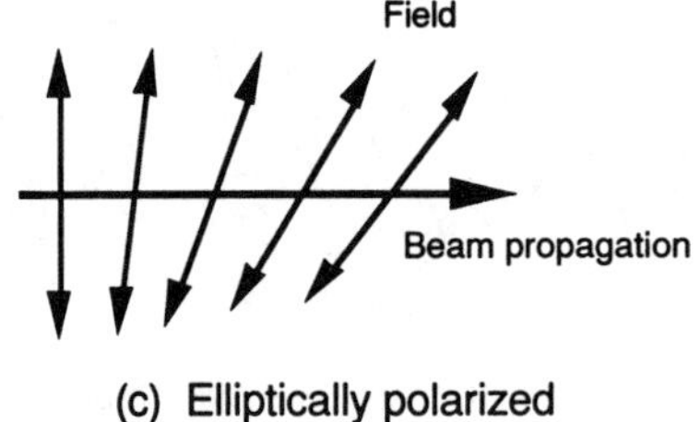

Figure 3-6 Linear, random, and elliptical polarization

Laser light may or may not be polarized, depending on the laser; but its polarization will effect many applications of lasers. Polarization is used in optical devices that are based on birefringence. A birefringent material splits incoming light into two linearly polarized parts that travel at different speeds in the material. The different speeds mean that the two parts of light (known as the extraordinary wave, or e-wave, and the ordinary wave, or o-wave) will represent different indexes of refraction. This difference can be combined with angles cut into the birefringent material to produce optical components that split light into parts. A common example is the polarizing beam splitter, or pbs. As shown in Figure 3-7, the pbs is made of two pyramids of birefringent material that are glued together with a special glue (usually glycerin or castor oil). Light entering the pbs is split into two parts. Because of the difference in index of refraction, one part undergoes total internal reflection at the intersection of the two components while the other passes through. The result is that the light is split into two parts which leave the pbs at right angles to each other.

Polarization can be produced by using filters or through reflection. Polarizing filters (such as Polaroid sheets) absorb light at one orientation while passing light that is oriented at right angles. As a result, unpolarized light passing through a filter will emerge plane polarized (and at a lower intensity since some light is absorbed). Circularly polarized light is produced by devices known as quarter wave plates. Quarter wave plates are birefringent and introduce a phase change of 90 degrees (or a quarter of a wave) between the e-wave and the o-wave. The result is that light emerges from the plate circularly polarized. Half wave plates (which introduce a phase change of 180 degrees, or half a wave) can be used to rotate linearly polarized light to a new angle of orientation.

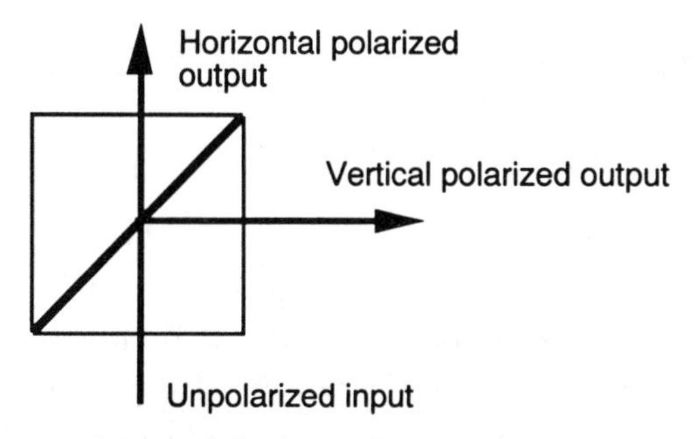

Figure 3-7 Polarizing beam splitter

Light reflected at a certain angle, known as Brewster's angle, will be linearly polarized. Brewster's angle is defined as that angle of incidence on a dielectric material where the transmittance for light with the electric field vector parallel to the plane of incidence is one. This is illustrated in Figure 3-8. Brewster's angle θ_b can be calculated by using Brewster's law:

$$\theta_b = \text{Tan}^{-1}\,(n_2 / n_1) \qquad \text{(Equation 3.3)}$$

where n_1 and n_2 are the refractive indices of the respective materials.

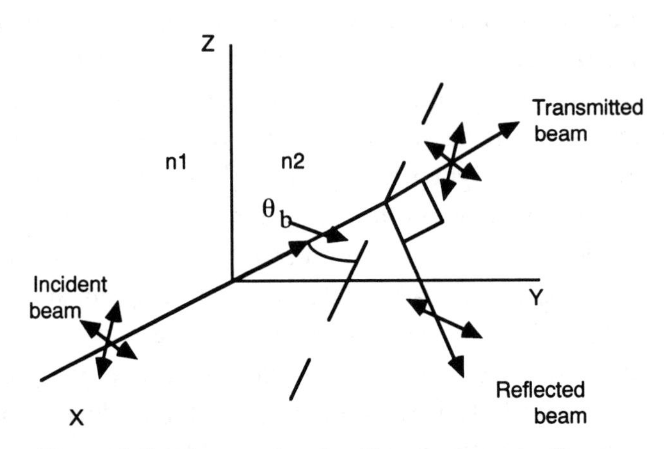

Figure 3-8 Diagram showing Brewster's angle, θ_b

3.2.3 Interference

The phase difference between two waves of light is an indication of the position of one wave relative to the other. Two waves that have a phase difference of zero degrees (in-phase light) are lined up so that peaks and valleys of the waves are in the same place at the same time (Figure 3-9a). Waves that have a phase difference of more than zero degrees, but less than 360 degrees (out-of-phase light) are misaligned. Waves that are 180 degrees out of phase (Figure 3-9b) are misaligned to the point that the peak of one wave is aligned with the valley of the other one.

Coherent light (light where the phase difference is constant) will exhibit an effect known as interference that depends on the phase of the waves. For constructive interference, waves that are in phase (no phase difference), and have the same amplitude, will combine to produce a wave that is equal to the sum of the individual waves. Waves that are

180 degrees out of phase, and have the same amplitude, will cancel each other out so that the net effect is that no light wave exists. This second effect is called destructive interference. It is the principle of interference that is used in many laser applications including holography and interferometery (see Chapter 8).

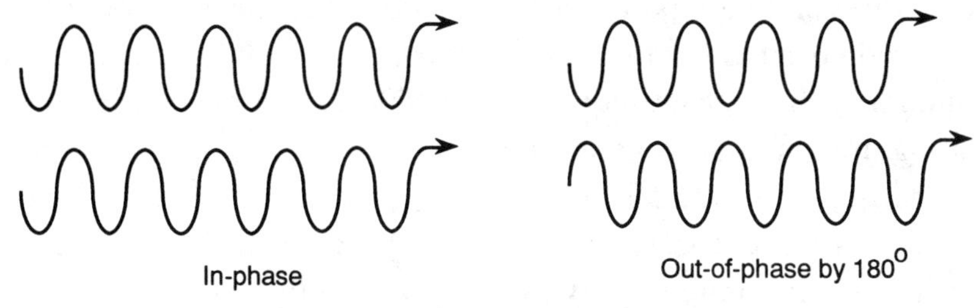

Figure 3-9 Wave phase relationships

3.3 Optical Components

3.3.1 High-Power Optics

The interaction of high-power laser radiation with any medium or optical components is often nonlinear and this imposes restrictions on the energy characteristics of high-power beams and their applications. Metal mirrors are often used with high-power lasers such as CO_2 lasers. These mirrors must be able to withstand high levels of radiation and have high thermal conductivity. Active cooling is often needed to reduce distortion and raise their damage threshold in high-power applications. Copper and molybdenum are commonly used for such mirrors; copper can withstand higher flux densities but molybdenum suffers less thermal distortion.

3.3.2 Power Optics

The applications of high-power lasers are related to the need for optical components capable of operating pulsed or cw mode. In pulsed mode, optical components should be able to withstand high peak-power loads, whereas in cw mode, they should be able to withstand continuous power radiation that generates a lot of heat.

All transparent optical components have limited optical strength because of self-damage caused by powerful light fluxes which occur on the surface and inside the material. Most conventional optical material cannot withstand high-power radiation without damage. Therefore, the design and construction of optical components should be characterized by minimum heat absorption and heat dissipation capabilities, while ensuring minimum distortion to the laser beam.

Mirrors are subjected to the greatest power loads in high-power systems. When uncooled mirrors are exposed to high energy fluxes, their lifetime is limited by overheating and deformation of reflecting surfaces. Metal mirrors are able to reduce these effects because they have better optical strength and temperature stability. They can also be cooled more effectively by heat sinks.

Cleanliness of optical surfaces is a critical factor in high-power optics. Defects in a mirror may be caused by inhomogeneities, inclusions, and surface contaminants. The task of producing defect-free metal mirrors is more difficult than for glass mirrors. Metal mirrors are softer and abrasive grains are easily imbedded in the surface during polishing.

Insulating films are used to protect reflecting metal layers from chemical interaction with the ambient medium, protect from mechanical damage, and increase mechanical strength of the coatings during the process of surface cleaning. Insulating materials used with high-power lasers should be characterized by low absorption at the working wavelength, chemical stability, high micro-hardness, and thermal expansion coefficient close to that of the substrate material.

3.3.3 Adaptive Optics

The distortions of the wave front of high-power beams can be removed by dynamic wavefront correction. Wavefront distortions occur when the beam passes through air and optical media. Simple adaptive optical systems can be adjusted to control focal length and wavefront inclinations in order to compensate for distortions.

There are two methods that can be used for adaptive correction. The first method using an optical system with wave front reversal is shown in Figure 3.10. The wavefront generated by a point source and its subsequent interaction with the medium are analyzed in order to optimize the beam qualities. A deformation mirror is used to deliberately introduce wavefront distortions which compensate exactly the distortions in the optical path. Essentially the wavefront distortions introduced into the beam are opposite in sign to the distortions acquired when the beam passed through the laser medium and air.

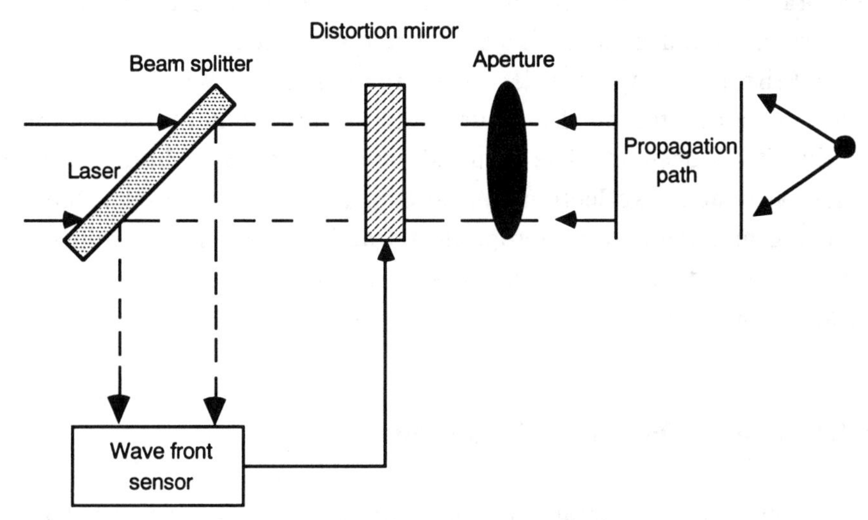

Figure 3.10 Adaptive optical system

In the second type of adaptive optical system, trial perturbations of the wave front are produced and an analysis is made of the intensity of a bright spot on a target viewed from a direction away from the path of the beam propagation. The results are used to determine what type of perturbations will optimize the propagation of a laser beam through an inhomogeneous medium.

The action of transmissive optics depends on the refraction of light passing through them. Refraction of light depends on the shape and refractive index of an optical component. Refractive index is a measure of the transmissive characteristics of the material that make up the optical component.

3.3.4 Laser Mirrors

Mirrors are used inside and outside a laser cavity. Standard mirrors are designed for long life and durability. Mirrors are chosen to provide low scattering, low temperature distortion, and high transmission properties. The mirrors most often used with lasers are evaporated coatings consisting of multiple layers of dielectric materials that are vacuum deposited on a transparent substrate.

Mirror coatings consist of alternating layers with a thickness equal to a quarter of the wavelength of the light of which high reflectivity is desired. The materials are alternately of high and low refractive index. Reflection can be adjusted to any desired value by choosing materials with appropriate refractive index and by adjusting the number of layers. Mirrors with up to 99.9% reflectivity are possible using multilayer dielectric materials.

3.3.5 Lens Defects and Aberrations

The best point image a lens produces is determined by what is called the ideal diffraction-limited case. In practice, a number of factors make this ideal impossible to achieve. Some of these factors are discussed below.

Spherical Aberration. Lenses have focusing imperfections that are present even in optically perfect components. A lens with a spherical surface does not bring parallel light rays entering it at different distances to the same focal point. This spreading out of the focus is serious for lenses with low focal ratio. Spherical aberration can be avoided by using lenses with nonspherical surfaces designed to avoid this problem or by restricting the entrance aperture.

Chromatic Aberration. Chromatic aberration is due to variations of refractive index with wavelength. Because of this, a lens brings light of different wavelengths to different focal points. However, lenses used with most laser systems have narrow spectral width which makes chromatic aberration insignificant.

Astigmatism. Light rays in a horizontal and vertical plane intersect at different points off the optical axis. The image of a point then appears either as an elongated ellipse or a line. Astigmatism is present in lenses if crossed lines do not appear as equally sharp images.

Curvature of Field. If the focal length of a lens were the same for all rays entering it, the focal or image surface would be spherical. Reducing the effects of field curvature requires that the region of interest in the focal plane be restricted to a smaller region about the optical axis.

3.3.6 Windows

A window is a flat transparent material that should ideally have no effect on light passing through it. Windows exist in optical systems to separate one physical environment from another. They are typically used where different ambient conditions are required in different parts of an optical system.

Gas laser tubes are often sealed with windows mounted at Brewster's angle. It transmits linearly polarized light without surface reflection losses. A Brewster's angle window does not eliminate light polarized in the orthogonal direction, but it introduces enough losses to make laser output strongly polarized.

Because all solids absorb some light passing through them, solid windows are vulnerable to optical damage when transmitting high-power beams. In order to avoid this, aerodynamic windows were developed to be used with very high power laser outputs.

General purpose windows are used because of high light transmission and surface qualities. Windows are used in the ultraviolet to near infrared wavelength ranges with surfaces polished to provide low scattering and prevent etalon effects. Etalon effects are changes in the optical path differences due to mechanical displacement or differences in refractive index.

3.3.7 Prisms

Prisms serve two functions in an optical system: (i) to disperse light by wavelength, and (ii) to redirect light without changing the beam size or relative alignment of the rays. Dispersive prisms rely on variations in refractive index with wavelength to refract different wavelengths at different angles to spread out the spectrum. In some optical systems, a slit is used to select a narrow range of wavelengths. Prisms can also be used in laser resonator cavities aligned so that only certain wavelengths will oscillate.

Beam redirecting prisms generally rely on total internal reflection to bend light, invert, and reverse images. Most are used with imaging systems rather than with lasers. The term prism also applies to polygonal blocks coated with reflective materials that function as mirrors. They reflect light from their outer surface so the light never enters the prism. Typically, such prisms rotate so the different faces sequentially scan a laser beam by reflection across another surface.

3.3.8 Transmissive Materials

The characteristics of optical components depend on the transmissive materials from which they are made. The wavelengths at which they are transparent depend on the internal energy structure of the material. Strong absorption occurs at wavelengths corresponding to energies at which the material can make a transition from its normal energy state to a higher one. The material is transparent at wavelengths corresponding to energy levels where there are no possible transitions. Transparencies differ among materials and none are transparent at wavelengths throughout the electromagnetic spectrum.

3.3.9 Ultraviolet Optics

Optical damage thresholds tend to be lower in the ultraviolet than in the visible or infrared wavelengths. Damage can occur in the material or at the surface, particularly to coatings used to enhance or reduce reflection. Material problems become increasingly severe at short uv wavelengths.

3.3.10 Infrared Optics

In many applications where the beam wavelength is in the far infrared, such as those produced by CO_2 lasers, typical glass or quartz optics cannot be used. Special infrared materials have been developed using alkali halides and some semiconductor materials. The two common features of infrared optical material are: (i) they are not typically transparent at visible wavelengths; (ii) many are hygroscopic and if left unprotected will slowly dissolve.

3.3.11 Filters and Coatings

Filters and coatings can alter the transmission characteristics of optical systems. Some filters are discrete components that derive their filtering characteristics from the nature of the optical material, but many are actually filtering coatings applied to plain transmissive optical substrates. Modern coatings can be applied in many ways, giving designers flexibility in selecting the properties of an optical system.

Spectral Filters. Many applications require selective transmission of certain wavelengths. Spectral filters are either based on physical mechanisms or optical functions. For laser applications, interference filters are commonly used to selectively transmit certain wavelengths and reflect others.

Spatial Filters. In laser applications, it is sometimes necessary to block the outer parts of a laser beam to remove stray light diffracted by dust and lens imperfections. This is done to reduce lens aberration effects and to improve wavefront quality. This function is performed by spatial filters which are essentially holes shaped to block unwanted portions of the beam.

3.3.12 Reflective Optics

Many mirrors have thin reflective coatings applied to substrates that have the desired flat or curved shape. Metal coatings are reflective over a broad range of wavelengths, while interference coatings are spectrally reflective in reflecting a limited range of wavelengths. Glass is a common substrate because of its good optical qualities and can be used in any spectral range.

BIBLIOGRAPHY

Akeel, Hadi. *Robots + Lasers = Accuracy, Flexibility*. Auburn Hills, MI: GMFanuc Robotics, 1991.

Hecht, Jeff. *The Laser Guidebook*. New York: McGraw-Hill, Inc., 1986.

Letokhov, V.S. and Ustinov, N.D. *Power Lasers and their Applications*. New York: Harwood Academic Publishers, 1983.

Luxon, James and Parker, David. *Industrial Lasers and their Applications*. Englewood Cliffs, NJ: Prentice Hall, Inc., 1985.

Luxon, J. Parker, D. and Plotkowski, P.D. *Lasers in Manufacturing*. Bedford, UK: IFS (Publications) Ltd. and Springer-Verlag, 1987.

Pinson, Lewis J. *Electro-Optics*. New York: John Wiley & Sons, Inc., 1985.

Ready, John F. *Industrial Application of Lasers*. New York: Academic Press, 1978.

Seippel, Robert G. *Optoelectronics for Technicians & Engineering*. Englewood Cliffs, NJ: Prentice Hall, Inc., 1989.

BIBLIOGRAPHY

4

LASER SYSTEMS AND COMPONENTS

Introduction

Besides the laser itself, most laser applications require other components and devices. The combination of these additional devices and components with the laser and its excitation source is referred to as a *laser system*. The parts of the laser system (other than the laser) can be divided into the broad categories of modulators and scanners, detectors, positioning systems, and optics.

Not all device types listed above are used with every laser, but the devices are common enough that they warrant some discussion. Chapter 4 deals with each of these (optics are also discussed in Chapter 3) by providing a discussion of the principles of operation, a description of common examples, and an explanation of how the device would be used in a laser system.

4.1 Modulators and Scanners

Modulators and scanners operate on the laser beam to change its direction or to alter its temporal characteristics (pulse the beam). The modulator may be housed inside the cavity for Q-switching and mode-locking, or outside the cavity for encoding data onto the beam. Scanners are used outside the cavity to direct the beam toward a specific location (or series of locations). The major types of modulators and scanners are mechanical, acousto-optic, and electro-optic.

4.1.1 Mechanical Scanners and Modulators

Principles of Operation. Mechanical scanners and modulators employ actual physical movement of a mirror, prism, or similar component to change the laser beam. The component is moved using an electric motor or through a galvanometer/coil arrangement. Mechanical scanners tend to be slow and difficult to control precisely, but they offer the advantage of relatively low price, durability, and simplicity.

Common mechanical scanners are galvanometer mirrors and rotating, multi-faceted mirrors. A common mechanical modulator is the beam chopper.

Common Examples. The galvanometer mirror works on the same principle as the d'Arsonval movement in an analog meter. A coil of wire mounted between the poles of a permanent magnet will rotate if a current is passed through it. Since the current causes a magnet field around the coil, the magnetic field of the permanent magnet will repel the coil and cause it to move. Varying the amount and direction of current in the coil will cause it to move different amounts and in different directions. A mirror mounted on the coil will move with it and can be used to reflect a laser beam in different directions.

Galvanometer mirrors offer the advantage of a large angle of deflection and little or no distortion of the laser beam. They are available in several different speeds and resolutions. Figure 4-1 shows a common galvanometer mirror. A combination of two such mirrors at right angles to each other can be used to position and scan the laser beam in two directions.

Rotating, multi-sided mirrors consist of a mirror with several sides that is rotated on a shaft. Each side of the mirror reflects the laser beam through an angle as it passes, and the next side of the mirror rotates the beam through the same angle. Using mirrors with more sides reduces the scanning angle but increases its speed. Speed can also be increased by rotating the mirror faster.

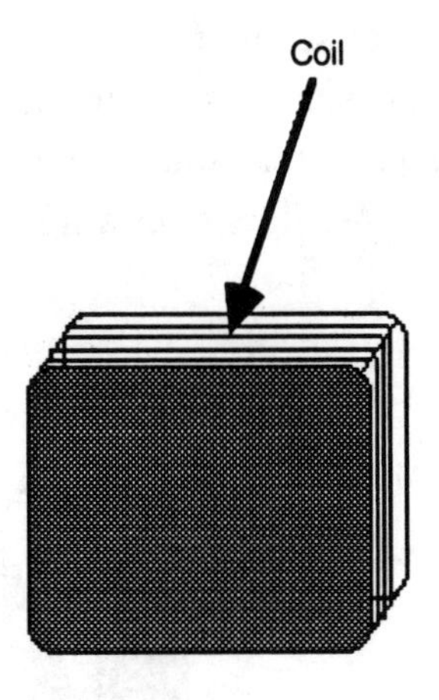

Figure 4-1 Galvanometer mirror

The disadvantage of a rotating mirror is that the laser beam can not be directed at a single point, but only scanned across an angle. Rotating mirrors are also relatively slow but are very simple to use and even to build. Figure 4-2 shows a typical rotating, multi-sided mirror.

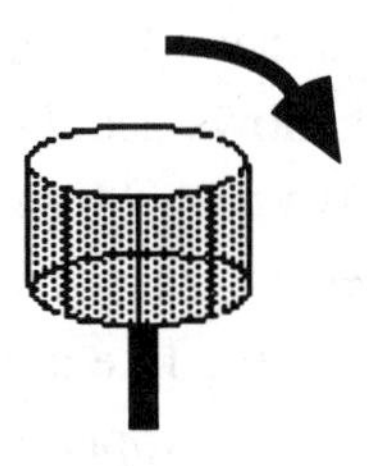

Figure 4-2 Rotating mirror

The light chopper is a modulator that is made up of a disk with fins cut into it, similar to a fan blade. When the disk is rotated, the fins block the path of the laser beam as they go by. The gaps in between the fins allow the beam to pass through. This rotating disk "chops" the laser beam as it revolves. The length of each chopped pulse is controlled by the size of the fins, and the frequency of the pulses is controlled by the speed of rotation.

Like all mechanical scanners and modulators, light choppers are slow but relatively inexpensive and simple. They are generally used with low or medium power beams, since higher power beams may damage the disk. Figure 4-3 illustrates a light chopper.

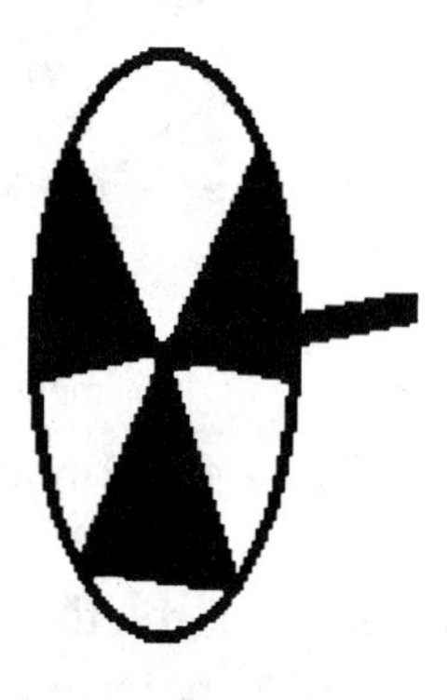

Figure 4-3 Light chopper

Common Applications. Mechanical scanners are used when a large range of movement is needed and high speed isn't necessary. A common application of a scanner like the galvanometer mirror is for a laser light show. Laser light shows use the special properties of the laser beam to create visual displays on a large scale (often accompanied by music). The scanner is used to trace a pattern with the beam from a visible light laser on some surface like a screen or a wall. By scanning rapidly enough, the traced pattern appears to be one solid line. Effects can be enhanced by adding smoke or steam in the beam path so that it too can be seen. Many commercial companies offer laser light shows for concerts and as stand-alone events. There are several permanent light show displays in the country.

Scanning the beam of a high-power laser on a surface can be used to engrave patterns on that surface. When the engraving only requires medium resolution on a small scale, a mechanical scanner can be used to position the beam. The scanner is often controlled by interfacing it with a computer that provides the appropriate current for each scanning position and allows the user to program individual position values or a model of the image to be engraved.

4.1.2 Electro-optic Modulators

Principles of Operation. The electro-optic effect found in some materials involves an interaction between an electric field and the polarization of light. In electro-optic materials, an applied electric field (voltage) will cause the material to become birefringent (see Chapter 3). This birefringence splits light passing through the material into two parts that travel at different speeds. When the light emerges from the other side of the material, its two parts will be recombined to form light having a different polarization. As shown in Figure 4-4, by carefully controlling the strength of the field and the size of the material, the electro-optic effect can be used to change the orientation of linearly polarized light.

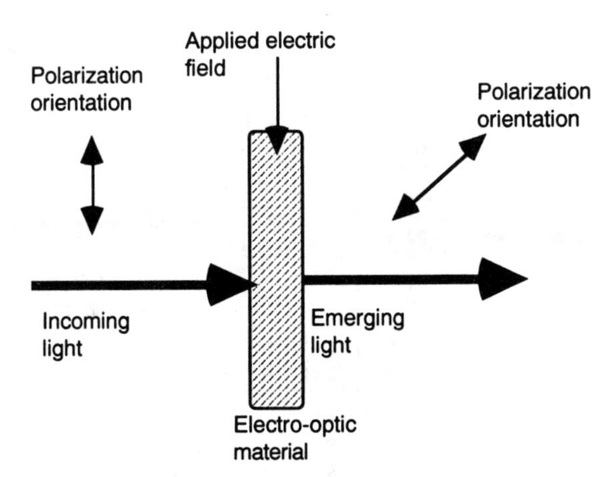

Figure 4-4 Electro-optic effect

Electro-optic modulators (or EOM's) combine the electro-optic effect with a combination of polarizing filters to modulate a laser beam.

The laser beam is passed through a polarizing filter (this first filter is not necessary if the beam is already linearly polarized) and then through the electro-optic material. Finally, the beam passes through another polarizing filter that is aligned with the first one. When the beam is passed through the first filter it becomes linearly polarized with a certain orientation. Passing through the electro-optic filter can have two possible effects. If the electric field is on, the orientation of the beam's polarization will be changed. If the field is off, the orientation will remain unchanged. When the beam reaches the final filter, it may be stopped if its orientation has been changed by the electro-optic material (since the filter only passes light of one orientation). The beam may pass through the final filter if its polarization is unchanged.

The electric field of the electro-optic modulator is turned off and on to produce pulses in the beam. The duration of the pulses is controlled by how long the field remains off, and the frequency is controlled by how rapidly the field is turned off and on in a given time span. Electro-optic modulators are very fast, but have the disadvantage of absorbing a relatively large amount of the laser beam as it passes through.

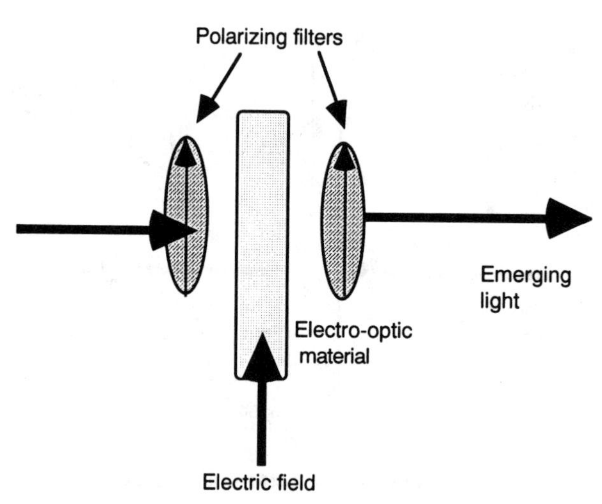

Figure 4-5 Electro-optic modulator

Common Examples. The Kerr cell is a common electro-optic modulator. The Kerr cell has a liquid as its electro-optic material and requires a relatively high voltage for its applied electric field. Also, the liquids used, such as nitrobenzene, are usually poisonous. For these reasons, the Pockels cell is more commonly used.

Pockels cells make use of a solid electro-optic material that is usually in crystal form. Common crystals are potassium dihydrogen phosphate (KDP) and ammonium dihydrogen phosphate (ADP). These materials require a voltage between 300 and 3000 volts and are useful for light ranging throughout the visible spectrum and into near infrared.

Common Applications. Electro-optic modulators are often used as Q-switches inside the laser cavity. Their high speeds make them useful, but the fact that they absorb a large percentage of the light that passes through them means they can only be used in lasers having a high gain. The ruby laser has enough gain to employ an electro-optic modulator. The modulator is inserted in the cavity between the ruby crystal and the output mirror. When the electric field is on, the modulator stops light from bouncing between the mirrors in the cavity and allows the crystal to build up a strong population inversion. When the field is turned off, the modulator allows light to pass and the beam reflects from both mirrors and is transmitted through the output coupler.

4.1.3 Acousto-Optic Modulators and Scanners

Principles of Operation. The acousto-optic effect is caused by sound waves in a crystal. If pressure is applied to a material it causes a change in that material's index of refraction. If the applied pressure is varied sinusoidally, the changes in the index of refraction will vary as well. In an acousto-optic device, high-frequency pressure changes (ultrasonic waves) are created in a crystal by vibrating its surface with a transducer. The waves in the crystal produce an effect similar to a diffraction grating (see Chapter 3). Light passing through the crystal will be split into two or more parts (or orders).

The angle of the split beam and the intensity of each part can be controlled by controlling the frequency and amplitude of the sound waves. Acousto-optic devices offer high speeds, but the deflection angles are not as large as a mechanical device and the beam is not completely directed or blocked off.

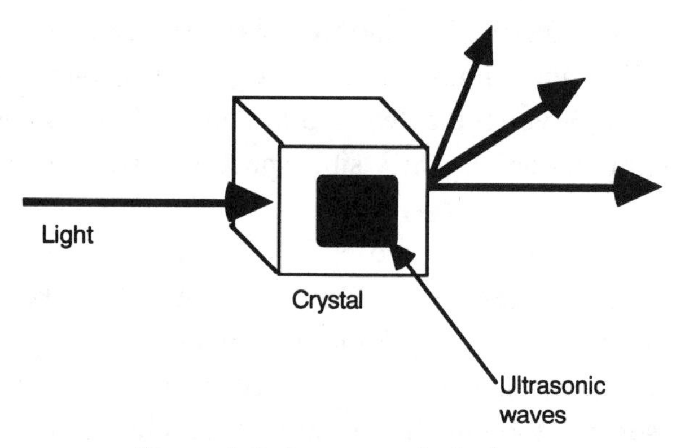

Figure 4-6 Acousto-optic device

Common Examples. The acousto-optic modulator (or AOM) is a common acousto-optic device. The crystal is frequently alpha iodic acid and the sound waves are created with a piezoelectric transducer. The transducer is driven by an RF driver which supplies high-frequency AC voltage which causes the transducer to vibrate.

The AOM can be used to modulate the laser beam by reducing the intensity of the part that leaves the crystal in the same direction as the original beam. Scanners use the part of the beam that is split at an angle to the original.

Common Applications. Acousto-optic modulators are often used as Q-switches when electro-optic devices cause too much loss. The Nd:YAG laser can be Q-switched with an AOM, and the frequency and duration of the beam pulse can be controlled by controlling the RF driver. The driver can be turned off to allow the laser to operate in the cw mode as well.

4.2 Detectors

Light detectors are used primarily to measure the amount of light in the laser beam. They may also be used for decoding information in a modulated beam or from a surface scanned by a beam. The types of detectors range from high speed/low beam power semiconductor devices to high beam power thermal detectors. Selection of the correct detector should take into account its responsiveness to light, wavelength sensitivity, speed, cost, and durability.

4.2.1 Semiconductor Detectors

Principles of Operation. Semiconductor detectors are based on the principle of a p-n junction diode (see Chapter 2). The junction of a semiconductor material with an excess of positive charges (p) with a semiconductor with an excess of negative charges (n) exhibits the photoconductive effect when a voltage is applied. When the diode is reverse biased (p of diode connected to negative side of supply and n of the diode connected to the positive side), there is a negligible amount of current flow. If the p-n junction is irradiated with light, electrons are freed from atoms and move through the circuit to produce current. An increase in light frees more electrons and causes an increase in current. Measuring the current in the circuit (or the voltage across the circuit load) will give an indication of the amount of light shining on the diode.

Common Examples. The two most common photodiode arrangements are the PIN photodiode and the avalanche photodiode. The design of the PIN photodiode increases the light sensitive area of the detector by adding an extra, *intrinsic*, layer of material between the p and the n layers. This intrinsic layer is not doped for extra charges but is a neutral material. Its presence causes an increase of the actual junction area that is the light sensitive region of the diode. The PIN photodiode is a low cost device that operates at a relatively low bias (5 to 20 volts) and is sensitive to the visible and infrared portions of the spectrum.

The avalanche photodiode (APD) is specially designed to detect small amounts of light. A large bias voltage is used to create a strong electric field across the p-n junction. This electric field accelerates electrons freed by the incoming light to the point where they free additional electrons from the surrounding material. These additional electrons may in turn free more electrons by the same process so that an incoming photon of light creates an avalanche of electrons. As a result, the APD produces a large current for a relatively small amount of light. Avalanche photodiodes are more expensive than the PIN photodiode and require a higher bias voltage that is well regulated.

Common Applications. The avalanche and the PIN photodiodes are used in detecting low-power laser beams such as those used in fiber-optic communications. Their spectral range and sensitivity means that they can be used for many communications and information processing applications. They are not suitable for detecting higher power beams such as those found in materials processing applications.

4.2.2 Thermal Detectors

When measuring laser beams that are high powered, the goal is generally to determine the amount of beam power (or energy) and the transverse mode of the beam. Detectors used in these applications incorporate a heat sensitive target which is heated by the beam. The temperature change in the target is measured and the beam power is calculated from this information.

Principles of Operation. Figure 4-7 shows a schematic diagram of a typical thermal detector system. The incoming beam is absorbed by the target which changes temperature. The temperature change in the target is measured and the beam power is calculated based on thermal properties of the target.

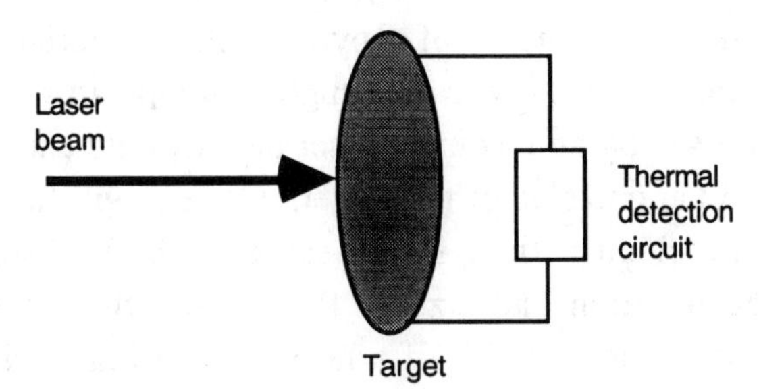

Figure 4-7 Typical thermal detector

Loss of heat by the target is controlled using insulation, and the detector is generally calibrated using a laser beam of known power. The thermal detection circuit can be one of two or three types depending on the application.

Common Examples. Thermal detectors used for continuous wave lasers are commonly called disk calorimeters. Pulsed laser detectors are known as joulemeters. The calorimeter is made up of a disk-shaped target whose temperature change is measured with a set of thermocouples that are linked together (known as a thermopile). Figure 4-8 shows the configuration of a disk calorimeter. The disk absorber acts as the target and may either be a surface absorber made of carbon, or a volume absorber made of a semi-transparent, dielectric material.

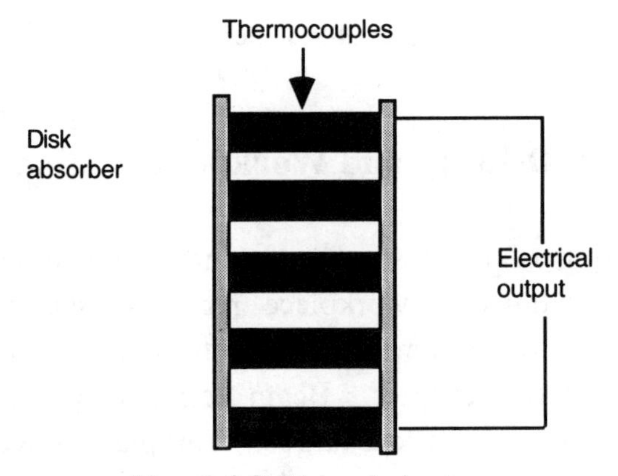

Figure 4-8 Disk calorimeter

The joulemeter consists of a pyrroelectric material which has an electric field that changes with a change in temperature. Increases in temperature caused by an incoming laser beam would cause a change in the electric field at one side of the target. Current will flow through the target until the electric field is the same on both sides again. By measuring the duration and size of the current flow, the joulemeter measures the duration and size of a laser pulse. Figure 4-9 shows the joulemeter arrangement.

Common Applications. Thermal detectors are used to measure the power or pulse energy of higher power lasers such as the Nd:YAG or the carbon dioxide laser. They are used when the beam powers are too great for measurement with a semiconductor detector.

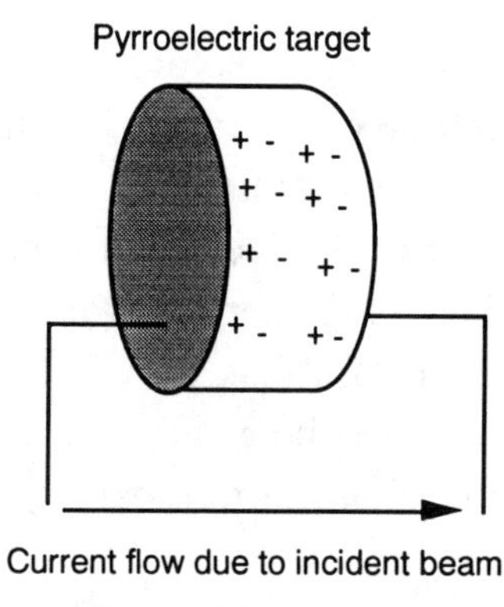

Figure 4-9 Joulemeter

4.3 Beam Delivery and Workpiece Motion Systems

Positioning of the laser beam (and in the case of materials processing applications, the workpiece) requires a special laser system. This system may have as some of its parts the components mentioned in other sections of this chapter. Beam delivery systems are used to position laser beams on a fixed target. Workpiece movement systems are used to position the workpiece under a fixed beam.

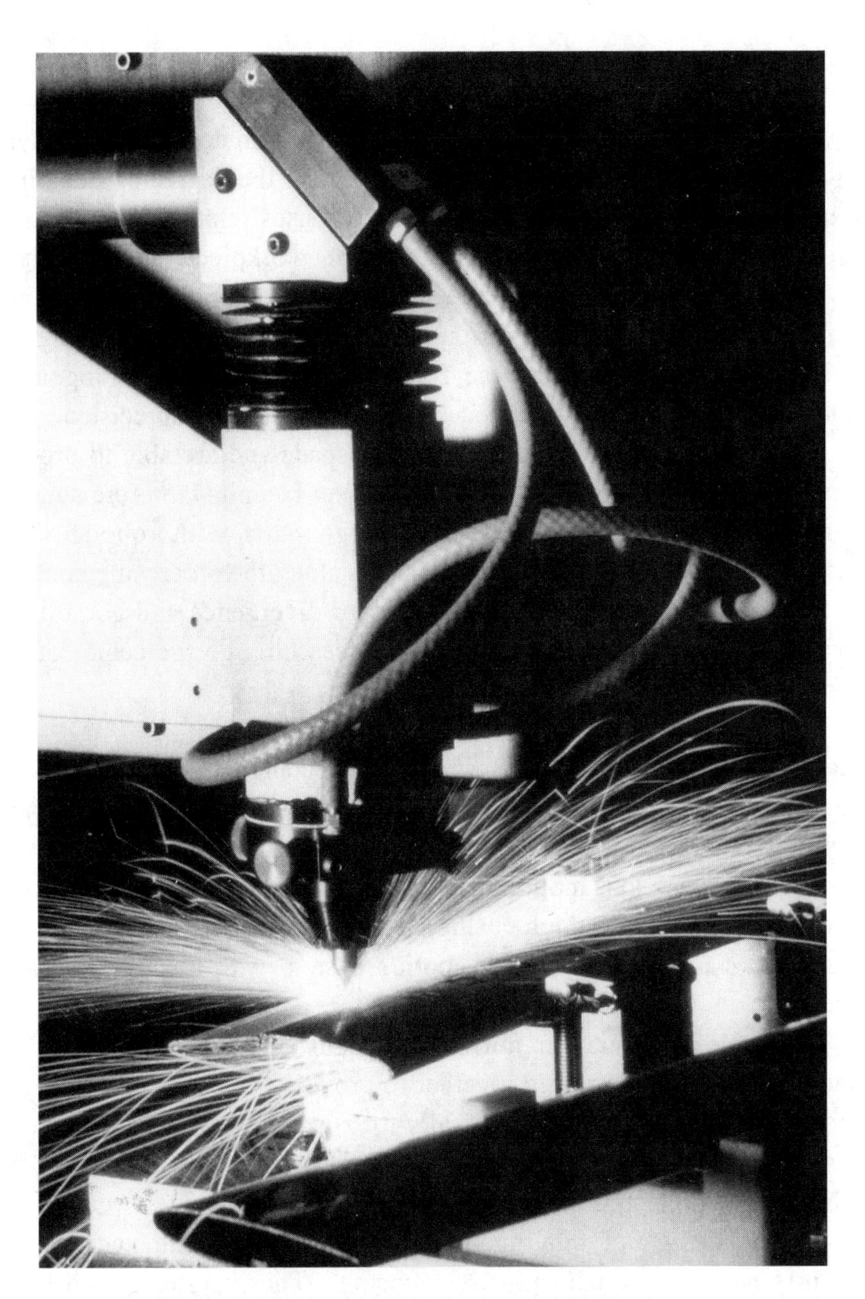

Figure 4-10 Beam positioning by an articulated arm
(*Courtesy of Coherent General, Inc.*)

4.3.1 Moving Beam Systems

The proper choice of a beam delivery system depends on the type of laser used, the nature of the application, and the degree of flexibility required. The moving beam configuration uses relative movement of the focused beam spot with respect to the workpiece. With a fixed position laser, the beam is deflected by one or more moving mirrors and a focusing unit. This ensures that the focused spot moves along the desired processing path on the fixed workpiece. This arrangement allows rapid positioning and processing speeds with high precision.

These systems use very little floor space and are able to process nearly all workpiece sizes. Moving the laser beam is therefore suitable for high-power laser processing of large parts with robots. One disadvantage is that the focus size changes along the processing contour. It also requires lasers with very low beam divergence and good beam axis stability to ensure that the beam passes through the center of the focusing lens.

Rectangular Moving Beam System. In a rectangular system, the beam can be moved in the x, y, and z-axis by numerical control. For small and low-power lasers, the entire laser head may be translated in the x and y directions. The z-axis motion may be carried out by control of a vertical slide or table to which the focusing assembly is attached. Figure 4-11 is a sketch of a rectangular beam motion system with a stationary laser head.

In this configuration, mirror m2 is translated to give the x motion, and both mirrors are moved together to provide the y-axis motion. The focusing assembly is moved vertically for z-axis motion. In some hybrid systems, the beam is moved in the x direction by moving mirror m2 while the workpiece is moved in the y-direction.

The design of moving beam systems is delicate because the mirrors have to maintain precise focusing. These systems tend to be more expensive and are generally only used for large, high-precision processing. But they offer many advantages including faster positioning and processing speeds, less stress and wear on the drive system, ability to process complex geometries, a stationary workpiece which reduces the need for fixturing, and quicker part changes.

Angular Beam Manipulation. For three-dimensional parts, a pure rectangular three-axis motion is often not sufficient. Some systems therefore utilize a combination of rectangular parts manipulation and angular beam manipulation. Large translational movements may be done by part movement while beam manipulation is used for smaller movements.

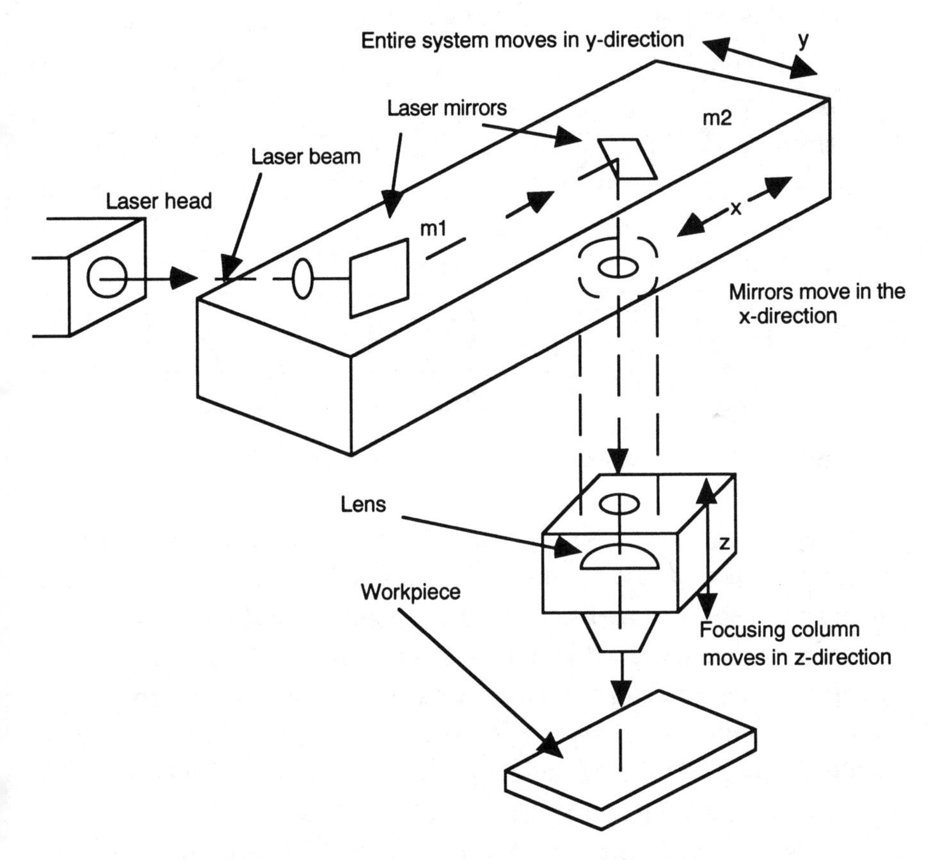

Figure 4-11 Rectangular beam motion system

Time-Sharing Systems. There are three ways of obtaining two or more beams from a single laser: time-sharing, beam splitting, and using a laser which outputs two or more beams directly. A laser beam is often time-shared between two or more workstations during production. This is particularly useful for cw lasers where the time taken for loading and unloading parts is a substantial fraction of the cycle time. One time-sharing arrangement is the in-line setup, with the laser elevated to eliminate having mirrors with upward horizontal projections. The first mirror is moveable to allow the beam to go on to the second workstation. But the mirrors have to be repositioned repeatedly with high accuracy in order to maintain alignment.

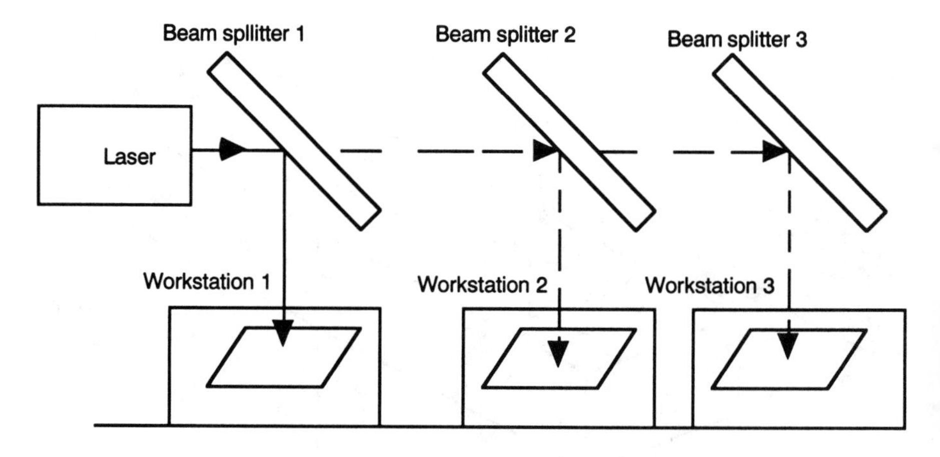

Figure 4-12 Beam splitting system

Beam Splitting. Beam splitting is sometimes a cost-effective way of using a high-power laser to do two or more jobs requiring less powers. The beam at several workstations is on simultaneously unless separate power dumps are designed into the system. Beam splitting systems must be correctly designed for the correct reflectance from each mirror. In the three workstation time-sharing systems shown in Figure 4-12, B.S_1 should reflect 33% of the incident power, B.S_2 should reflect 50% (1/2 of 66.7%), and the final mirror should reflect 100%.

Lasers which produce more than one output beam are an alternative to beam splitting. Fiber-optics can also be used in low-power applications to deliver multiple beams to several locations at the same time.

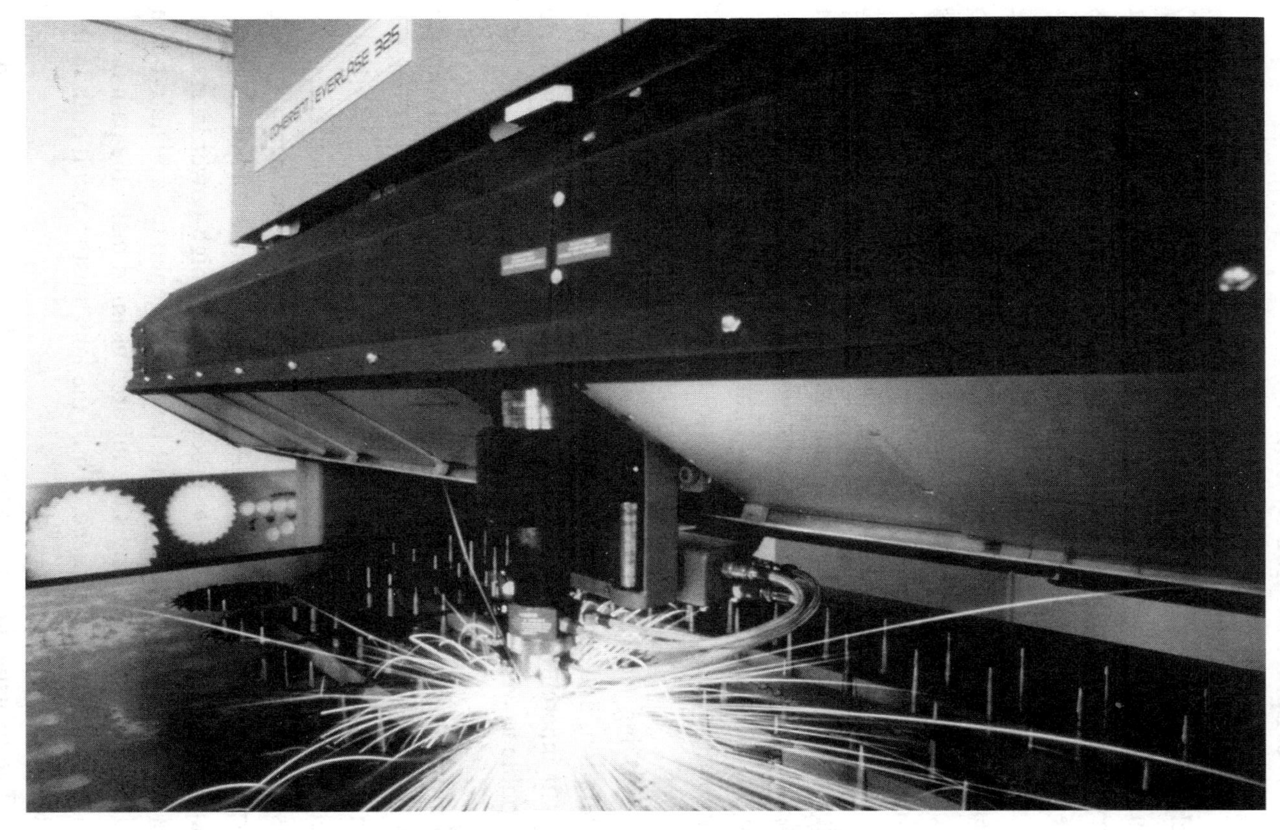

Figure 4-13 A laser cutting system using a CNC table
(*Courtesy of Coherent General, Inc.*)

4.3.2 Workpiece Motion Systems

Many materials processing applications use a fixed-beam system which utilizes parts handling systems to move the workpiece. Parts may be manually or automatically loaded and then rotated, indexed, or otherwise automatically translated. For precision and circular parts processing, focus adjustments remain fixed during processing. For non-precision parts, some form of focusing axis control is used. These systems are suitable for large cutting and welding laser systems to process small sizes of material. Processing of thicker and larger sizes requires more floor space.

The efficiency of many applications is often determined by the ability and speed of the materials handling system which moves the part into position. Some moving systems employ an x-y axis table. Tables are light, fast, accurate, and can be controlled by computerized inputs. Contouring speed of tables can also be controlled to very precise positions.

Moving workpiece systems impose problems with acceleration, deceleration, and maneuvering large masses in two dimensions. This makes it inherently slower than moving optics, less precise, and more susceptible to wear on the drive mechanism.

Common Example—Moving Workpiece System. A typical moving workpiece system is illustrated schematically in Figure 4-14. First, the beam coming out horizontally from a high-power laser is vertically directed by a beam bending mirror. The deflected beam then enters the focusing unit where a focusing lens concentrates the beam on the workpiece. The focusing unit also contains a gas nozzle adjacent to the workpiece for cutting and other processes. Most high-power lasers also use a low-power He-Ne alignment laser that generates a visible beam coaxial to the path of the invisible infrared beam to make the path of the beam visible on the workpiece. Thus, the lens must transmit both in the visible and infrared wavelengths.

The focusing unit as a whole can usually be moved up and down (normal to the workpiece surface) to ensure the unit has the appropriate separation from the workpiece. The separation is usually only a fraction of a millimeter to avoid expansion of the cutting-gas flow. The focusing unit must also be lifted for the loading and unloading of workpieces, which is done pneumatically or by some other technique for high speed. The workpiece itself can be moved by a z-axis coordinate table that moves or allows the workpiece to move across it.

Below the gas nozzle the table has a hole that opens into a box connected to an exhaust system. The box acts to absorb the remainder of the beam coming out of the lower side of the workpiece, collect molten debris, and exhaust the vapors produced during cutting.

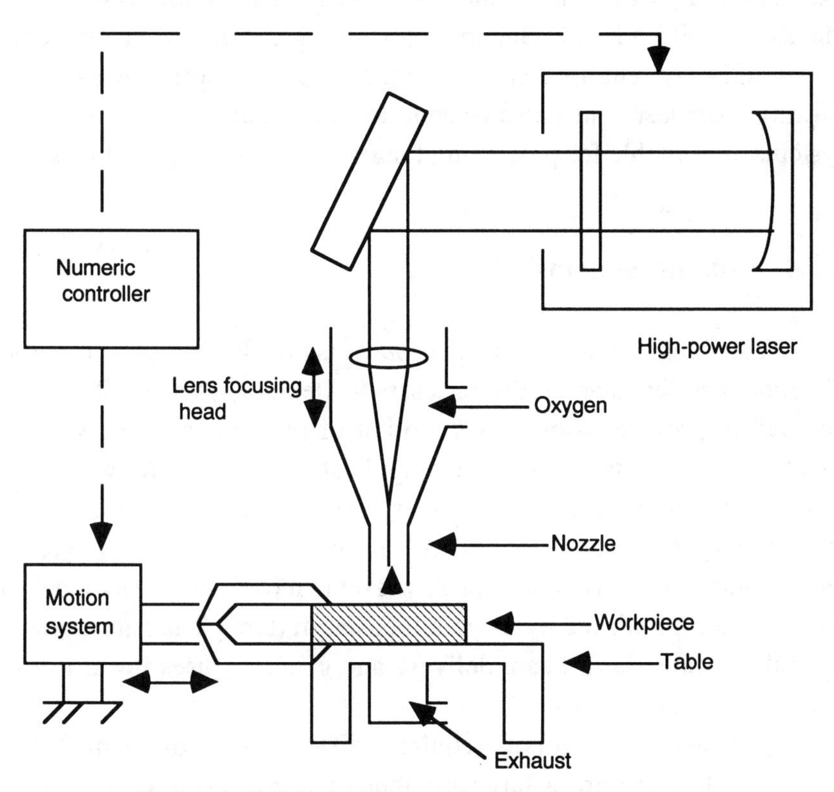

Figure 4-14 Principal layout of a laser cutting system

All the units are controlled by a central numerical controller. Thus, all the following operations are initiated and controlled by a computer: the cutting process, movement of the focusing unit, movement of the workpiece, and control of the laser power level. Appropriate circuits and software serve to avoid incorrect sequencing during the process. Special devices such as interlock switches that avoid displacement of parts serve to ensure safe-use high-power laser beams.

4.3.3 Hybrid Systems

This approach moves the laser head in one axis and the workpiece in another. Hybrid systems save on costs and have less complex drives because both the beam and the workpiece move in single straight-line axes only. However, coordinating movement between both traveling members is difficult. Moving the workpiece generally lowers processing speed and may require a special fixturing setup to prevent parts from shifting. The laser must also be shut down to load/unload parts. Hybrid systems are suitable for processing long narrow parts such as tubes.

4.3.4 Robotic Systems

The integration of lasers and robots is mainly due to the flexibility of robots and the adaptability of lasers to flexible systems. Robots can be used to provide 5- or 6-axis motion of parts beneath a fixed laser beam for some material processing applications. There are two types of robotic systems used for beam manipulation: the gantry robot and the articulated arm robot. A gantry robot is basically an overhead rectangular motion system with x, y, z-axis movement. Angular beam motion is accomplished by using a focusing fixture. The gantry robot is natural for direct laser beam delivery and generally uses fewer mirrors, thus reducing power loss.

Articulated arm robots require a different type of beam delivery system. They require a large number of mirrors (ten or more). To minimize the number of mirrors needed, efforts are directed at designing compact lasers with sufficient power to be placed on the shoulder of the robot. Some dedicated robots are designed so that the beam can be directed through the robot's arm.

4.4 Optical Components

Optical components play an integral part in shaping and positioning the laser beam. The principles of optics as well as some typical optical devices are outlined in Chapter 3. This section concentrates on particular optics that are commonly used in laser systems.

Folding Mirrors. Folding mirrors are used in most industrial CO_2 laser systems to reduce overall length of the laser to a fraction of the cavity length. They are also used to determine the polarization of the output beam if the angle of incidence is large. Folding mirrors are usually made from coated silicon because of its optical stability under thermal load. Most intracavity mirrors have protective and reflectivity enhanced coatings.

Brewster Windows. Brewster and vacuum windows are generally used in low-power lasers because thermal instability limits their use in high-power systems. Windows are used in gas lasers to separate the discharge volume from the surrounding atmosphere. They must be thick enough to withstand pressure differences and must also be made of homogeneous material in order to preserve the wavefront of the transmitted radiation.

Brewster windows are inclined at a very high angle (Brewster's angle) which has the property of transmitting most of the p-polarization component and reflecting most of the s-polarization (see Chapter 3). They can therefore be used as intracavity polarizers to determine the plane of polarization. They are usually rectangular or elliptical and are always uncoated.

Beam Expanders. Beam expanders are used in material processing laser systems for several reasons. They may be used to increase beam size for the reduction of power density in order to minimize damage to optics. Beam expanders are also used to reduce divergence and may result in smaller focused spot size. Beam expanders or collimators may be used for spatial filtering of the beam, which may produce improved power density at the focused spot.

Zero Phase-Shift Mirrors. Polarization insensitive materials have been developed to eliminate the problems polarization may cause in some applications. Mirrors with special coatings are able to produce equal reflectance for both components of polarization for a specific angle of incidence. Such mirrors are used inside and outside the resonator cavity.

Multiple Mirrors. Moving beam systems are becoming more widely accepted in industry due to the adaptability of robotic systems. Such systems may incorporate more than ten mirrors which generate the need for coatings with high reflectivity and polarization preserving properties.

Beam Splitters. Beam splitters can be used to generate several output beams that can be used to do simultaneous processing. A beam splitter is coated to reflect a definite proportion of incident light and transmit the rest. Standard beam splitters have reflection/transmission ratios of 50:50, 30:70, and 10:90. These ratios are achieved by polarizing the beam either horizontally or vertically with respect to the direction the beam will have after splitting. The beam first hits the partial-reflecting coated side of the mirrors, the second side is anti-reflection coated. These optics are edge-mounted to allow both reflected and transmitted beams to propagate.

There is typically a 20%-30% difference in the performance of the two polarization states. Thus, it is imperative to specify the polarization state of the incident beam with respect to the geometry of the beam splitter surface placement. If the polarization of the incident beam is not polarized in the s or p direction, the polarization of the reflected beam will be complicated. Because polarization insensitive beam splitters are difficult to manufacture, incident beams are usually polarized in the s or p plane of the optic.

Focusing Element. Convex lenses or reflecting parabolic concave mirrors are used to focus the laser beam as it exits the beam delivery system. Focusing lenses must be antireflection coated to reduce surface reflections. Many applications such as cutting require the highest power density attainable in order to maximize processing speed. Short focal length single meniscus lenses designed for minimum spherical aberration are used for focusing operations.

Beam Benders. Beam benders are used to deflect the beam several times on its way to the work space in a typical system. Beam benders consist of two cylindrical, hollow conduits whose axes intersect and incline by equal angles to an external mirror's surface. When the beam enters from one conduit aperture along its axis, it reflects directly along the axis of the other conduit, and changes its direction by an angle equal to the angle subtended between the two conduit axes.

Circular Polarizers. Polarizers are used to avoid undesirable polarization changes in complex optical systems. Circular polarizers convert linear polarized beams into circular polarized beams which are desired for many materials processing applications. A circular polarizer using four mirrors is shown in Figure 4-14. Birefringent coatings on the mirrors alter the polarization state of a linear polarized beam.

Two of the four mirrors have 1/8 wavelength coatings which produce a 1/4 wavelength phase-shift in one component of the electric field relative to the component at a right angle to it. If the electric field of a linear polarized light beam entering such a device is properly oriented, the emergent output beam will be circularly polarized.

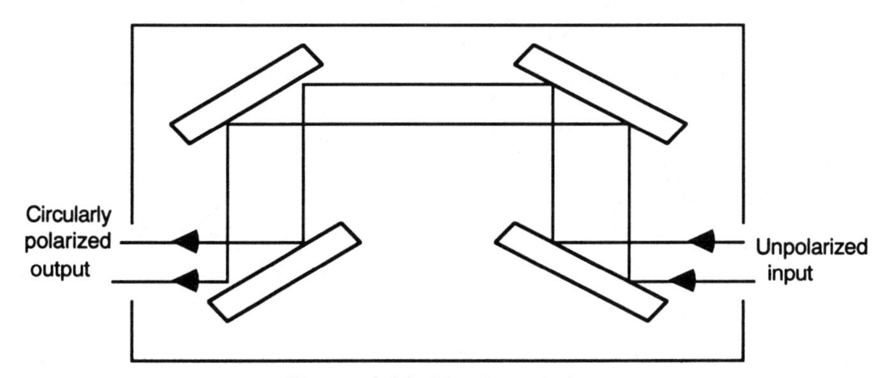

Figure 4-14 Circular polarizer

Conduits. As a beam travels through the laser system it is necessary to protect the human eye from the beam, as well as protect the beam from airborne particles obstructing its path and contributing to power loss. Straight line conduits extend between beam benders. Their internal surfaces are usually opaque antireflection coated to absorb peripheral beam radiations that would otherwise affect beam polarization.

Optical Joints. These allow the beam to deflect and rotate about its axis of entry. The most common is the right-angle rotary joint which permits the beam to rotate in a plane perpendicular to its direction. Other optical joint configurations rotate the beam in a conical mode. Optical joints must have high degrees of accuracies, particularly where the beam travels over long distances.

Linear optical joints allow the beam bending location to change along the laser beam axis. These joints are versatile because they can be coupled with a rotary optical joint, allowing beam manipulation over an extensive work space with freedom of multiple orientation.

Beam Shutter. The laser beam energy must be switched on and off to control its application at the workstation. This is not convenient for some types of lasers such as those with d-c discharge, because of the time needed to initiate and propagate the laser at each startup. Beam shutters are used to dump available laser energy into an energy absorber that interrupts the beam path or deflects the beam into a heat sink. Systems that deflect the beam generally have faster response time than those directly interrupting the beam path.

BIBLIOGRAPHY

Akeel, Hadi. *Robots + Lasers = Accuracy, Flexibility*. Auburn Hills, MI: GMFanuc Robotics, 1991.

Facts about: Laser Cutting. Norway: AGA Sweden and Institute for Product Development, 1991.

Franan, Dennis and Shelmire, Gary. "Measuring Laser Output—Calorimeter or Joulemeter?" *Laser & Optronics*, September, 1991.

Hecht, Jeff. *The Laser Guidebook*. New York: McGraw-Hill, Inc., 1986.

Kloczkowski, Robert L. *A Comparison of Laser Cutting Systems*. Cincinnati: Cincinnati Incorporated, 1986.

Lasers. New York: Coherent, Inc., McGraw-Hill Book Co., 1980.

Laser Technology for Effective Parts Making. Cincinnati: Cincinnati Incorporated, 1991.

Letokhov, V.S. and Ustinov, N.D. *Power Lasers and their Applications*. New York: Harwood Academic Publishers, 1983.

Luxon, James. "Optics for Materials Processing." *The Industrial Laser Annual Handbook*. Tulsa: Penwell Publishing Co., 1986. ed. David Belforte and Morris Levitt.

Luxon, James T. and Parker, David E. *Industrial Lasers and their Applications*. Englewood Cliffs, NJ: Prentice Hall, Inc., 1985.

Luxon, J. Parker, D. and Plotkowski, P.D. *Lasers in Manufacturing*. Bedford, U.K.: IFS (Publications) Ltd. and Springer-Verlag, 1987.

O'Shea, Donald. *Elements of Modern Optical Design*. New York: John Wiley & Sons, Inc., 1985.

Pinson, Lewis J. *Electro-Optics*. New York: John Wiley & Sons, Inc., 1985.

Ready, John F. *Industrial Application of Lasers*. New York: Academic Press, 1978.

Schuocker, Dieter. "Laser Cutting," *The Industrial Laser Annual Handbook*. Tulsa: Penwell Publishing Co., 1986. ed. David Belforte and Morris Levitt.

Seippel, Robert G. *Optoelectronics for Technicians & Engineering*. Englewood Cliffs, NJ: Prentice Hall, Inc., 1989.

Welsh, Michael. "Optics for Materials Processing CO_2 Lasers." *The Industrial Laser Annual Handbook*. Tulsa: Penwell Publishing Co., 1986. ed. David Belforte and Morris Levitt.

Unit II

APPLICATIONS OF LASERS

Like the laser itself, the applications of lasers involve a wide range of fields. Many applications are developmental or only recently implemented, and although models exist for describing them, there is still much trial and error in the implementation. For many applications, there are established companies that provide a good deal of support in designing and implementing the appropriate laser system. Unit II provides a discussion of the applications of lasers in several different fields. The intent is to provide a good basic understanding of how and why an application works without spending much time on engineering considerations such as design and theoretical (and mathematical) modeling.

Chapter 5 covers the diverse field of laser materials processing including welding, cutting, drilling and marking. A discussion of beam parameters and material parameters and how they relate begins the chapter. Workpiece fixturing, beam delivery and engineering considerations end it.

Chapter 6 combines the fields of communications and information processing. An introduction to communications is included and a special emphasis is placed on fiber optics as the most common communications application. Bar-code systems, optical storage of audio and computer data, and laser printing are the topics included under information processing.

Chapter 7 looks at medical applications and especially at therapeutic applications where the laser is used in surgery and treatment. A look at the interaction between the beam and tissue is included as well an overview of the basic ways the laser is used. Specific treatment procedures are also discussed.

Chapter 8 covers sensing and measurement. Such topics as interferometry, holography, and fiber optic sensors are discussed.

Again, please consider safety when working with lasers. Refer to Appendix C for an in depth discussion.

5

LASERS IN MATERIALS PROCESSING

Introduction

Materials processing is a general term that covers common processes such as welding, cutting, and drilling that affect the physical properties of a material. The concentrated energy of higher power lasers makes them useful tools for many materials processing applications. Since laser beams require no physical contact with the material, they have the advantage over more conventional methods involving mechanical drills or saws. It is also possible to deliver a laser beam to remote locations and to incorporate lasers with automated machinery.

Lasers are currently used in several areas of materials processing. The most common applications include welding, drilling, cutting, and engraving. Materials ranging from metals to plastics to ceramics have been successfully processed with lasers. Lasers are often used in the assembly and fabrication of electronic components, the production of aerospace parts, and engraving of a wide range of products and materials.

Carbon dioxide (CO_2) lasers have long been the workhorse of laser materials processing, but solid-state lasers such as Nd:YAG and Nd:glass are playing an increasing role. Ruby and excimer lasers have also carved their own niche in the field.

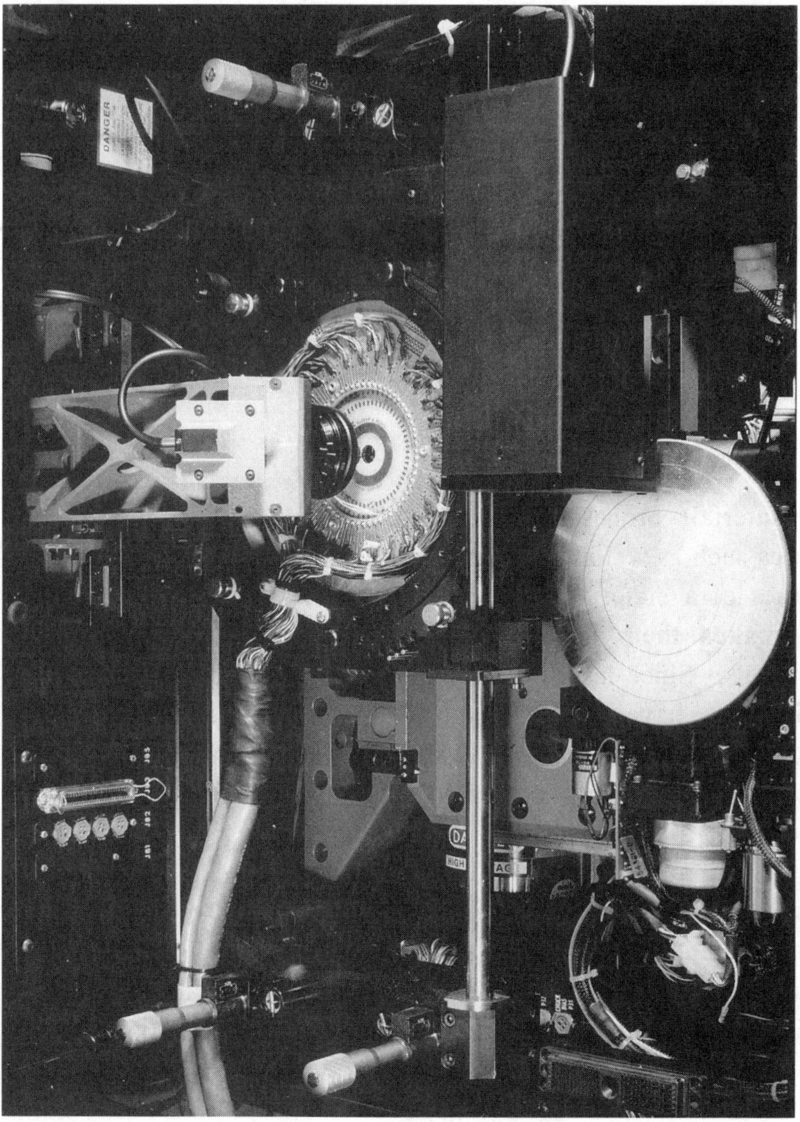

Figure 5-1 A typical laser processing system
(Courtesy of Electro Scientific Industries, Inc.)

5.1 Parameters that Affect the Process

Understanding the role of a laser in a materials processing application requires a close look at the properties of both the laser beam and the material. The size and shape of the laser beam along with its power and energy will greatly affect the outcome of a process. Material properties such as reflectivity and thermal parameters are also important. We will begin our discussion by examining each parameter individually.

5.1.1 Laser Beam Parameters

The main laser beam parameters for materials processing are listed in Table 5-1. Each property has its own level of importance and its own potential for adjustability. Beam parameters are not isolated values, but are related to each other. The value of one will affect the values of the others.

Table 5-1 Laser Beam Parameters
Beam Power/Energy
Beam Diameter
Power Density
Transverse Mode
Wavelength
Pulse Shape and Duration
Polarization

Power. The *power* of a continuous wave laser beam (or *energy* of a pulsed beam) is the most obvious beam parameter that affects a process. Materials processing generally involves an increase of temperature in order to melt (welding), vaporize (cutting and drilling), or change the physical properties (heat treating) of a material. Higher power levels mean that this temperature change can be accomplished more rapidly.

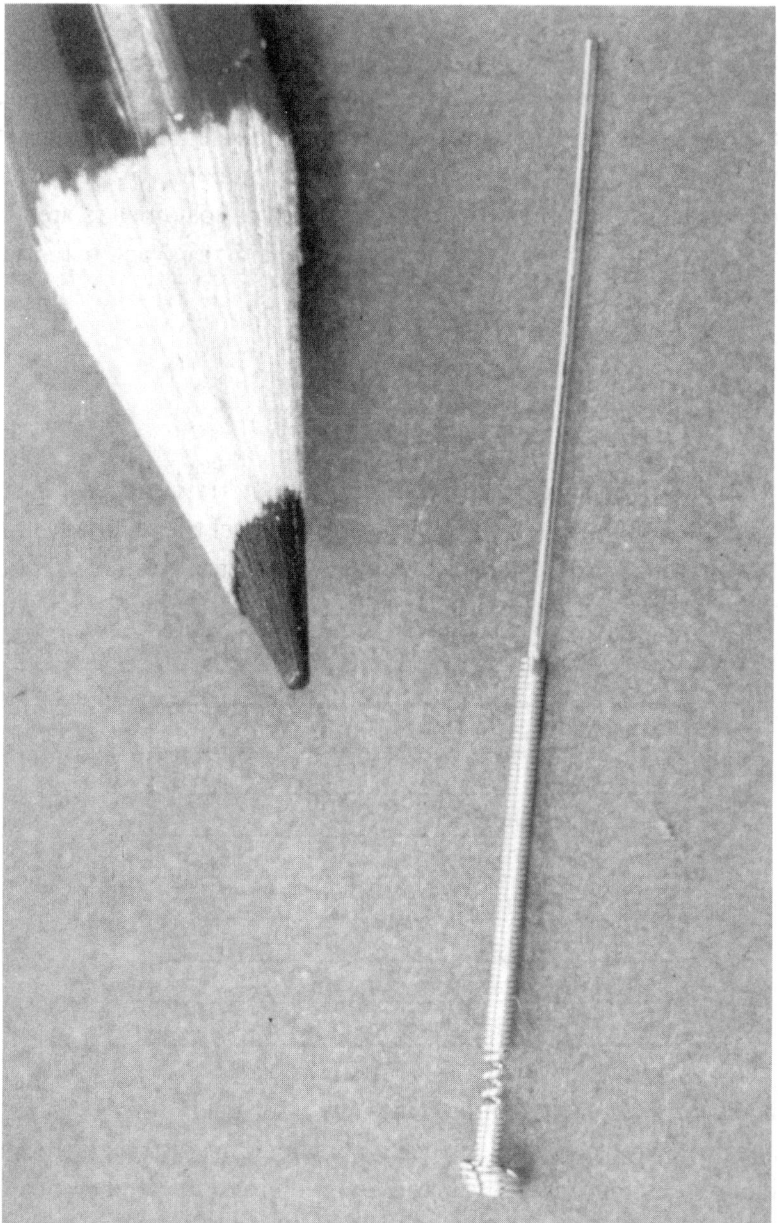

Figure 5-2 Small-scale laser processing
(*Courtesy of Coherent General, Inc.*)

However, an excessive amount of power can result in undesirable effects. As an example, laser welding requires melting the material. Too much power could cause the material to vaporize, leaving craters in the weld. Refer to Chapter 1 for more discussion about laser power and energy.

Determining the proper power levels for a particular application begins with considering the thermal and reflective properties of the material and applying that knowledge to the temperature change required. The information provided by these theoretical considerations gives a good starting point for the application. Optimum power levels can then be determined experimentally by making adjustments to the power and observing the quality of the outcome.

Beam Diameter. The size of the laser beam (expressed as *beam diameter* or spot size; see Chapter 1) governs the area of the material affected. In most applications, the laser beam is confined to a small, well-defined area. In drilling, the depth, diameter, and shape of the hole depend on the size of the beam. Beam diameter is also important in terms of the *power density* of the laser. Power density is defined as the power per cross sectional area of the beam.

$$P_d = P / A \qquad \text{(Equation 5.1)}$$

where

P_d = power density
P = power, and
A = area.

Smaller beam diameters mean higher power densities. Higher power densities indicate more laser power in a smaller area.

Wavelength. Laser beam *wavelength* is an important consideration but not one that is easily adjustable. Materials will absorb different amounts of light at different wavelengths. The laser beam's wavelength also places a theoretical limit on how small a beam can be focused, and will dictate what types of optics can be used in the system. Laser wavelengths at high powers are predominantly in the infrared region, although visible and UV beams are also available. Some wavelength alterations can be made through frequency doubling or other non-linear effects. Generally, lack of absorption at a particular wavelength is compensated for by increasing the power density.

Transverse Mode. Optimum laser processing comes from the gaussian beam profile of a TEM_{00} output (see Chapter 1). Gaussian profiles focus more efficiently and provide a predictable power distribution. Higher powered lasers often output several transverse modes. Their beams don't follow the gaussian model exactly, but do obey it to the first approximation. The actual beam diameter of an unfocused beam can be determined by scanning the beam with a detector and recording the power at regular intervals. A graph of the resulting data will give a profile of the beam. Passing the beam through a calibrated aperture and determining the transmission ratio is another method for determining diameter. A rough approximation of beam diameter can also be found by irradiating a heat-sensitive target and measuring the resulting heat-affected zone. Refer to Chapter 4 for more information about determining beam properties.

Pulse Duration. Lasers that produce pulsed outputs are used in many materials processing applications. The *duration of each pulse* will govern the total amount of power delivered to the material. The frequency of the pulses affects how the thermal properties of the material will change after each beam interaction. In many cases it is suitable to apply a pulse that begins at a high power and then decays exponentially. Such pulse ramping overcomes the initial reflectivity of the material and then operates at a lower temperature once the material has changed states.

5.1.2 Material Properties

Material properties (listed in Table 5-2) are largely unadjustable. Many materials, because of their thermal properties, are not suited for laser applications. The absorption of a material also limits its

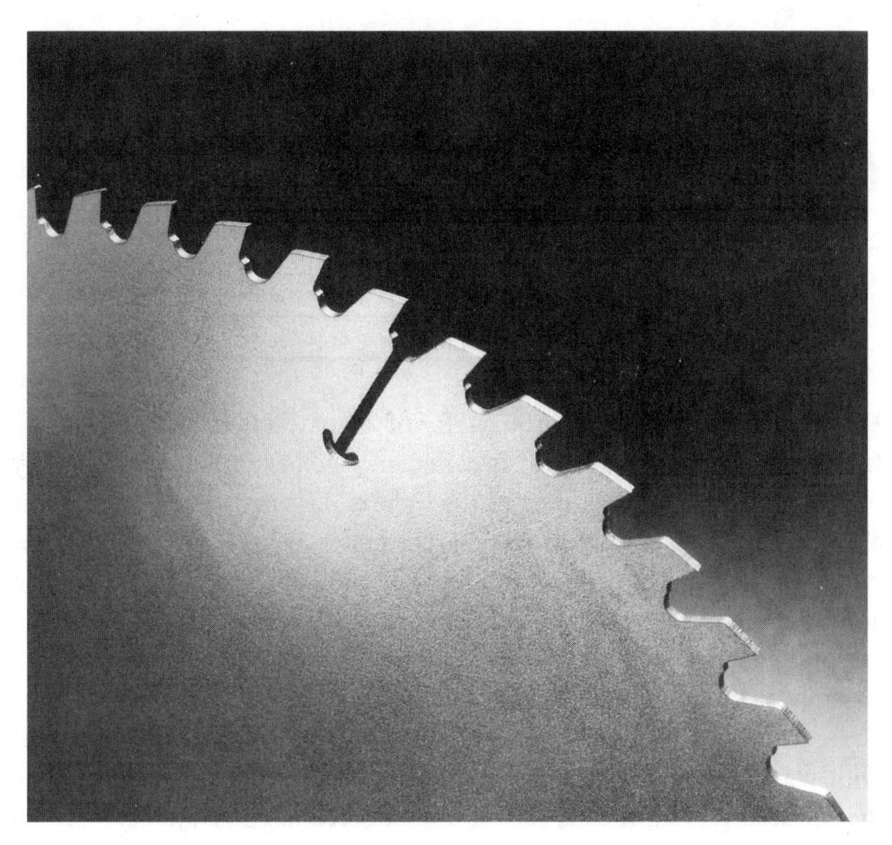

Figure 5-3 Example of a laser-beam cut
(*Courtesy of Cincinnati Incorporated*)

suitability, although this can be overcome by modifying the surface condition.

Table 5-2 Material Properties
Reflectivity
Surface Condition
Specific Heat
Thermal Diffusivity

Reflectivity. The *reflectivity*, R, of a material is defined as the fraction of incident light that is reflected. For example, a reflectivity of 0.80 means that 80 percent of the light is reflected, and 20 percent is absorbed (or transmitted in transparent materials). Reflectivity varies with wavelength, angle of incidence, and surface condition. In addition, the reflectivity will also change as the material changes states. A solid material will reflect differently than the same material in a gaseous or liquid state.

The reflectivity of metals (in the solid state) generally increases with wavelength. Since the majority of high-power lasers operate in the infrared region, metals reflect a high percentage of the beam, often more than 90%. Since wavelength is determined by the type of laser used, beam power levels must be increased to overcome this reflection. The angle of incidence is usually fixed at 90 degrees in a materials processing application.

Surface Condition. The *surface condition* of a material can greatly affect the reflectivity. Rough surfaces generally absorb more of the beam, but can also lead to irregularities in reflectivity and thermal effects. Smoother surfaces will be more uniformly affected but will also cause higher reflection. In many cases the surface of the material is preconditioned to improve the absorption. Experimental data can be used to determine ideal surface condition. When the application does not allow changing the surface condition, beam parameters such as power density must be adjusted to compensate.

Changes in state (solid to liquid, liquid to gas) of the material can cause complex absorption/reflection affects. In applications where material is removed by vaporization (such as cutting and drilling), the vaporized material will form a cloud or plume that changes the absorption. In cases where the plume reduces the absorption of the beam, it is often removed with a stream of pressurized gas. This gas can also serve to aid in the chemical reaction that changes the state of the material.

Specific Heat. The thermal properties of a material are used to predict the effects of an incident laser beam. The amount of energy required to increase the temperature of a certain amount of material is determined by its *specific heat*, c, expressed in joules or calories per gram degrees Celsius. The energy required is given by the equation

$$H = mc\Delta T \qquad \text{(Equation 5.2)}$$

where

H = energy required
m = mass of the material
c = specific heat, and
ΔT = temperature change.

H is sometimes referred to as the enthalpy of the material.

In addition to temperature change, energy is required to change the state of a material. The amount of energy to change states from solid to liquid is given by the latent heat of fusion. Energy required to vaporize a material is given by the latent heat of vaporization. Determining the amount of energy required to perform a certain process requires adding the amount of energy required to change temperatures to melting or boiling point and adding the energy required to change states. This total is the amount of energy that must be absorbed by the material. The actual energy required of the laser beam is much higher because of reflection losses.

Thermal Diffusivity. When the temperature of a material is increased, the heat does not remain stationary but flows toward the cooler parts of the material. The rate that the heat flows will determine how long the laser beam must be applied to the material and how much of the material will be affected. *Thermal diffusivity* is the material property that characterizes heat flow. The diffusivity involves the rate of heat flow in a material (thermal conductivity, K) and the specific heat. It is defined by the equation

$$\text{diffusivity} = K / pc \qquad \text{(Equation 5.3)}$$

where

K = conductivity
p = density, and
c = specific heat.

High thermal diffusivity means the heat will flow rapidly. The laser beam must be applied for a longer time period to compensate for higher diffusivity values.

5.2 System Requirements

Materials processing requires more than just the laser and the material. The system also includes optics for focusing and shaping the beam, a method of delivering the beam to the material, some way to mount the material (commonly called the workpiece) in place, and a way to move the beam relative to the material, or the material relative to the beam. Some of these topics are covered in detail in Chapter 4, and principles behind beam focusing and beam delivery are also discussed in Chapter 3. This section will be confined to discussing these principles in the context of materials processing.

Table 5-3 System Requirements
Beam Focusing
Beam Delivery
Workpiece Fixtures and Positioning

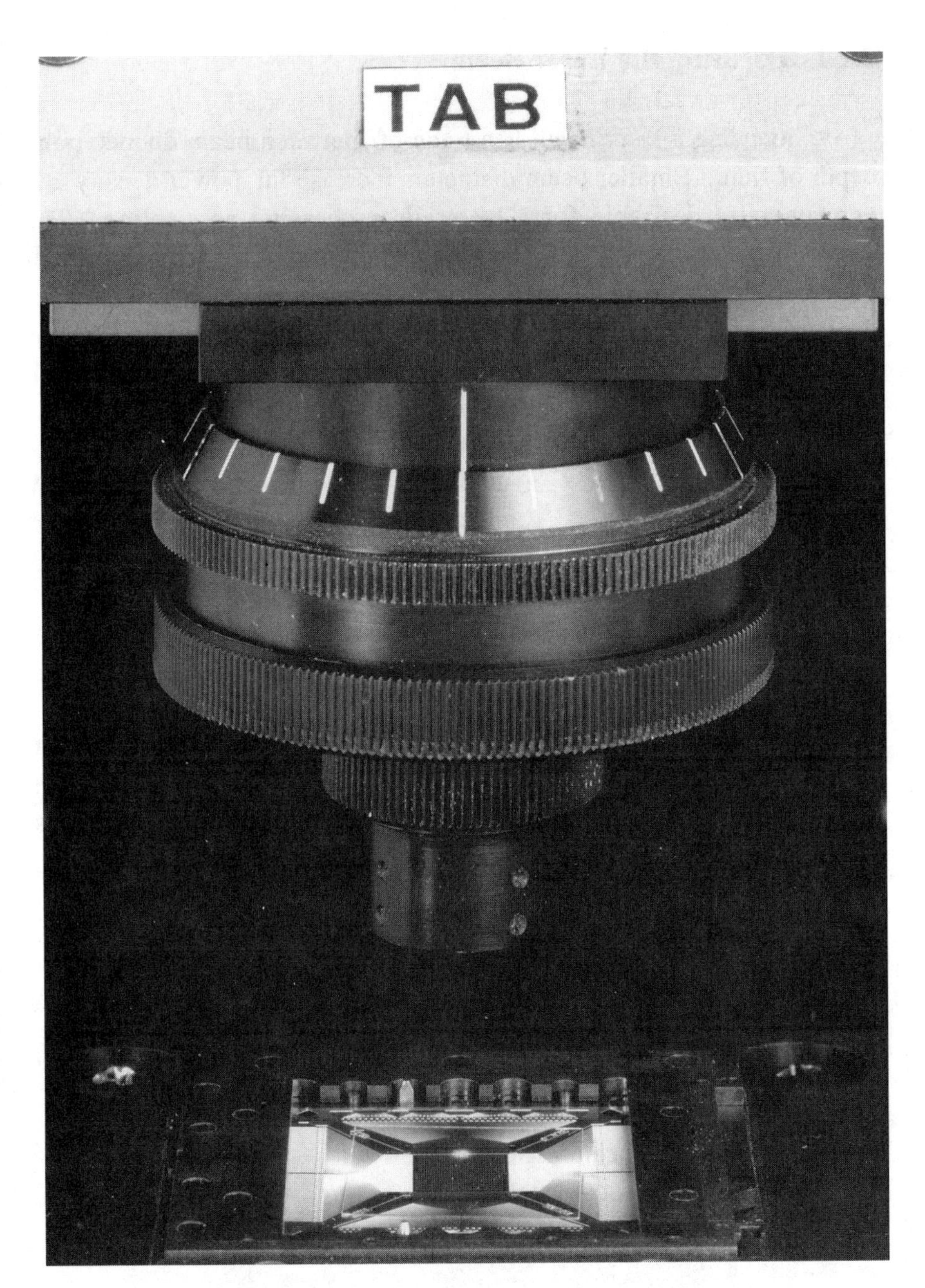

Figure 5-4 Focusing optics for an Nd:YAG laser
(*Courtesy of Electro Scientific Industries, Inc.*)

5.2.1 Focusing the Laser Beam

Focusing a laser beam is a trade-off between beam diameter and depth of field. Smaller beam diameters increase the power density and are generally desirable for a materials processing application. The distance into the material that the beam remains at its minimum diameter, known as depth of field, grows shorter as the beam diameter decreases. Long depths of field may be required for processes (such as drilling or thick welds) that require a deep penetration of the material. Beam diameter and depth of field are related by the equation

$$z = 0.32\pi w^2 / \lambda \qquad \text{(Equation 5.4)}$$

where

z = depth of field
w = beam spot size, and
λ = wavelength.

The depth of field, z, is defined as the point where the beam diameter is increased by 5%. Since the thermal effects of the beam can extend beyond the depth of field and depend on the thermal properties, actual penetration should be determined experimentally.

The diameter of the focused beam is governed by the focal length of the optics used and the divergence of beam. Focal length, divergence, and beam diameter are related by the equation

$$d = f\theta \qquad \text{(Equation 5.5)}$$

where

d = beam diameter
f = focal length, and
θ = divergence.

The beam divergence can be reduced through collimation (see Chapter 4), but this also increases the diameter so that it must be reduced even further. In many cases the added effects of collimating the beam before focusing it are negligible when compared to the benefits of a smaller beam diameter.

5.2.2 Beam Delivery

For lasers that operate in the far infrared or ultraviolet regions of the spectrum, beam delivery is limited to direct irradiation of the material or directing the beam through a combination of mirrors. Using a large number of mirrors to route the beam through a complex path (as in the articulated arm of a robot) leads to a large number of alignment problems. Alignment is generally accomplished using a low-power, visible laser beam that is coaxial to the beam used in the application. This eliminates the hazards of aligning the invisible and dangerous beam of the working laser. Changes in mirror position through vibrations during the operation of the laser make it necessary to realign the delivery mechanism at regular intervals. Direct irradiation is a simpler approach to beam delivery, but it can be difficult especially when working with a large laser cavity or a workpiece that is difficult to access or has multiple areas that need to be irradiated. Most systems operate with a small number of mirrors that deliver the beam to the workpiece which is often positioned with numerically controlled fixtures.

The development of fiber optics has created a new realm of beam delivery for lasers that operate in the near infrared or visible portion of the spectrum. Fiber-optic beam delivery has an advantage over mirrors because alignment is minimum. The fiber can be routed through complex areas and positioned close to the workpiece. The laser can even be located in a remote location. A single laser beam can be multiplexed into several fibers and routed to separate workpieces simultaneously. Fiber-optic beam delivery has been successfully used with multi-kilowatt lasers with no adverse affects. In fact, the fiber has the beneficial effect of evenly distributing the beam power in a gaussian profile. See Chapter 1 for more details on gaussian profiles. Chapter 6 discusses the principles of optical fiber.

5.2.3 Fixturing and Positioning the Material

The workpiece needs to be securely mounted so that it will not change its position relative to the beam during the process (an exception is when the workpiece is purposely moved to deliver the beam to different areas). Since most processes are applied to several workpieces sequentially, the fixture needs to consistently hold each workpiece in the same position. Several methods have been used to hold a workpiece (see Table 5.4). Choosing the proper fixture involves considering the size, shape, and weight of the workpiece as well as the method of beam delivery involved. For instance, vacuum suction cups may be well suited for holding lightweight materials like textiles or thin metallic materials, while hydraulic vices may be required for heavier materials. In cases where the workpiece is an unusual size or shape, it may require a customized fixture that could incorporate one of the methods listed in Table 5-4.

Table 5-4 Workpiece Fixturing
Vacuum/Suction Devices
Hydraulic Vices
Pneumatic Vices
Mechanical Vices
Fixed Guides and Clamps

In cases where it is not practical to position the laser beam at several different spots on a workpiece, the workpiece can be moved while the beam is held stationary. Moving the workpiece involves the well-developed technology of numerical control. The workpiece is fixtured to a table that is translated by the movement of electronic motors. These motors can be precisely positioned by means of an electronic controller that is often interfaced with a computer. These computer numerically controlled (CNC) systems allow the user to program complex patterns for the workpiece to follow. It is not unusual to use a CNC system that operates in three dimensions. Addition of rotation can add an additional dimension to the system.

The development of computer aided design (CAD) software has allowed the development of the pattern in a drafting environment. This pattern can then be transferred to the CNC controller electronically.

5.3 Processing Application: Laser Welding

Welding involves joining two or more pieces by filling the space between them with a molten material that acts as a bond when it solidifies. Laser welding uses the beam to melt the edges of the two pieces at the gap and allowing those edges to fuse and form the weld. Since laser welding needs only to melt the material, the beam power density must be controlled so that the materials do not vaporize. Laser welding has been successfully performed in different types of metals as well as plastics. Welds have been made in large applications as well as small electronic components and circuit boards.

5.3.1 Laser Welding Fundamentals

The laser beam forms a weld by penetrating the material and forming a cavity called the *keyhole*. As the beam travels along the weld, the molten material fills in this gap and forms the bond. The vapors generated by this interaction are often removed using a stream of inert gas that is coaxial to the beam. The speed at which the laser beam moves along the weld will affect the depth of the weld as well. Higher speeds will result in less depth because the beam does not have enough time to penetrate. Increases in power density will cause increases in weld depth up to the point where the density causes the material to vaporize instead of melt. The size of the gap between the pieces will also affect the weld. Since the laser relies on the melted edges of the material to form the weld, these edges need to be very close together. Several different types of bonds can be formed with a laser weld. Some of the simplest are illustrated in Figure 5-5. In each case, the laser beam has to be directed at the proper part of the bond to form a weld.

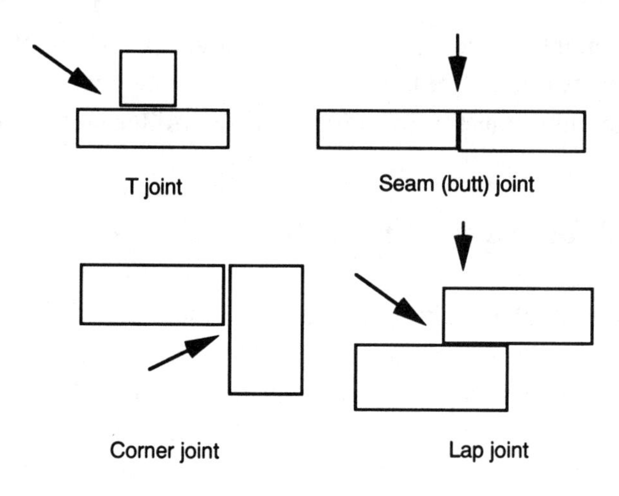

Figure 5-5 Weld types

5.3.2 Example—Welding Stainless Steel with a CO_2 laser

As an example of laser welding, consider welding two stainless steel plates in a butt joint. The steel is 0.75 mm thick, and the weld is meant to be 8 cm long. The plates are smooth along the edges and on the surface. The initial selection of the proper laser, power levels, beam size, welding speeds, and positioning and delivery system is an engineering decision. Technical methods of maintenance, troubleshooting, and operation will be required once the system is chosen.

Engineering Considerations. Selecting the proper laser for the welding process involves many practical considerations in terms of initial and operating costs, availability, and other factors that are unique to each company. We will confine ourselves to the more technical considerations involved in selecting a laser. The number of lasers capable of providing the required beam power are limited to molecular lasers (such as the carbon dioxide laser) and solid-state lasers (such as Nd:YAG). The reflectivity of stainless steel is virtually equal for any these lasers (roughly 0.98) since they primarily operate in the

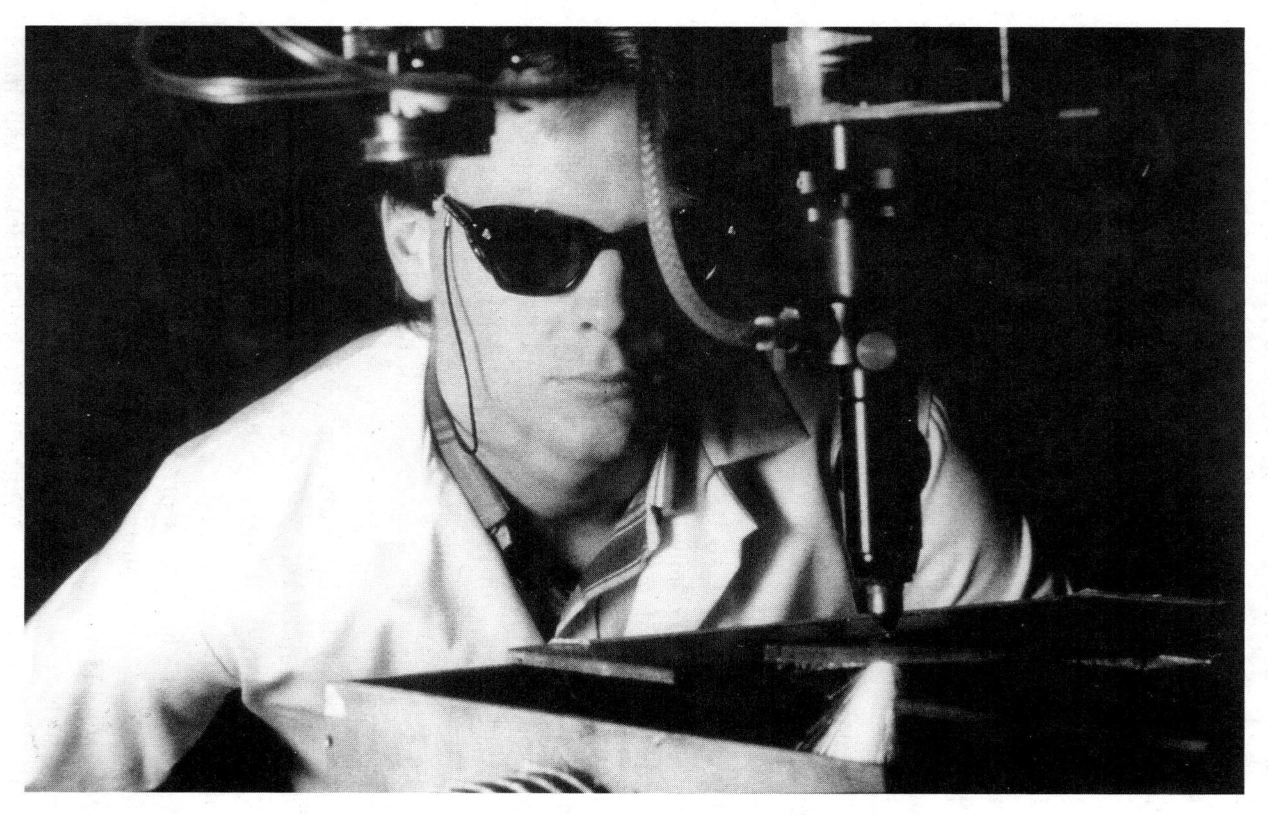

Figure 5-6 Technician monitoring a laser-cutting operation
(*Courtesy of Edison Welding Institute*)

infrared. With that in mind, let us consider an Nd:YAG laser operating 1064 nm as the laser we will use. We must now consider the amount of beam power required, as well as the beam diameter and welding speed.

Calculating the required beam power can be a fairly complex process. The melting depth is the primary factor that governs the amount of power that the material should absorb. For our application, the melting depth will be equal to the plate thickness (0.75 mm). Calculating the amount of energy required to melt the material involves considering the thermodynamics of the system. The laser beam will increase the temperature of the material closest to it first, and the heat flow through the material will determine how quickly the rest of the material will change temperature. Since the heat flows in three dimensions, and part of the material will melt and change its thermal properties before the rest, the mathematical model for melting is not trivial. Fortunately, experimental data for many materials is readily available. This data gives us a reasonable starting point for determining the beam power. For materials where data is unavailable or in applications where a more complete picture of the process is desired, the engineer must resort to the mathematical model. For 304 stainless steel, we will take the power required to be 0.075 kW (75 watts) applied at a weld speed of 1 cm/s.

Since 98% of the laser beam will be reflected by the steel, the beam power must be high enough to compensate. If 75 watts of beam power is required, then approximately 750 watts must be applied.

Initial setup of the system requires adjusting beam power and welding speeds to produce the best weld. Care should be taken to keep the material parameters (surface condition and the gap between the parts) constant during this procedure. The beam power should be maximized and kept constant while the welding speeds are adjusted through a wide range of values. By comparing the results, the optimum weld speed can be determined.

During operation, changes in beam parameters and material parameters can cause changes in the weld quality. A reduction in beam power would cause a loss of weld depth or quality. Beam power should be monitored closely, preferably continuously by installing an on-line detector (see Chapter 4 for more on determining and adjusting beam power).

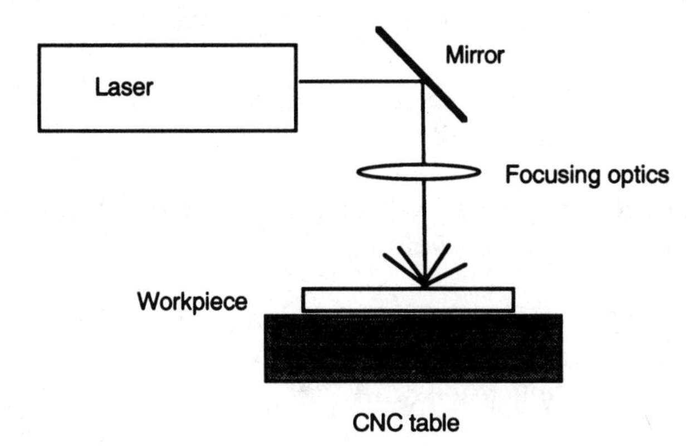

Figure 5-7 Welding carbon steel

BIBLIOGRAPHY

Belforte and Levitt, eds. "Material Processing Data and Guidelines," *The Industrial Laser Annual Handbook, 1990 Edition*. Tulsa: Penwell Books, 1990.

Charschan, S.S. ed. *Lasers in Industry*. Toledo: Laser Institute of America, 1972.

Introduction to Lasers. Waco, TX: Center for Occupational Research and Development, 1987.

Kim, T.H., Albright, C.E., and Chiang, S.L. "The Energy Transfer Efficiency in Laser Welding Process" *Journal of Laser Applications LIA,* vol. 2 January/February, 1990.

Mueller, R.E., Duley, W.W., MacLean, S., Garneau, M., Tryggvason, B. and Evans, W.F.J. "Laser Welding of Plastics in Low and High Gravity Environments" *Journal of Laser Applications LIA,* vol. 1 July, 1989.

Ohse, Roland. "Laser Application in Material Science and Technology: Materials Processing, Surface Modification, and High Temperature Property Measurement" *The Industrial Laser Annual Handbook, 1990 Edition*. Tulsa: Penwell Books, 1990.

Sercel, Jeffrey and Sowada, Ulrich. "Why Excimer Lasers Excel in Marking" *Lasers & Optronics* September, 1988.

Shukov, George and Smith, Al. "Michromachining with Excimer Lasers" *Lasers & Optronics* September, 1988.

6

LASERS IN INFORMATION PROCESSING AND COMMUNICATIONS

Introduction

The use of light in information processing and communication has increased rapidly with the advent of semiconductor light sources and especially the laser diode (or semiconductor laser). Light offers several advantages over other technologies. As a communications carrier, light has a higher frequency than radio or TV waves and modulated electrical signals in copper wire. In optical storage devices, there is no physical contact with the medium, which means no wear or losses from frequent use. The unique properties of *laser* light (such as monochromaticity and coherence) have created new areas of information manipulation that were not possible before.

The use of lasers in information processing and communications is widely varied. Some applications remain in the development stage, while others are confined to limited or specialized areas. This chapter will focus on the more common applications, and fiber-optic communication and optical storage media are discussed in detail. Information manipulation in the areas of barcode technology and laser printers are discussed briefly. An introduction to communications is provided as background for discussions on fiber-optics.

6.1 Fundamentals of Communications

Communication is the process of transferring information from one point to another. There are three basic steps to communication—*encoding*, *transmission*, and *decoding*. Consider the example of communication via a telephone system. The information or data (in this case a person's words) is encoded by the telephone onto an electronic signal (*carrier*). The carrier passes through copper wires, which we call the *medium*, to the telephone at the other end. The receiving telephone decodes the data by reversing the process used at the transmitting end. Methods for encoding/decoding and types of carriers and media vary from one communication system to the next.

6.1.1 Encoding and Decoding

The major methods of encoding are divided into *digital* and *analog*. Digital encoding imposes digital data onto a carrier by representing it as a series of pulses. In the simplest case, a pulse would represent the binary bit, 1, while the absence of a pulse would represent the bit, 0. Figure 6-1 shows a set of binary information imposed on a carrier. The duration, shape, and peak value of the pulses are important since they will be used by the receiving end to identify pulses and separate one pulse from another.

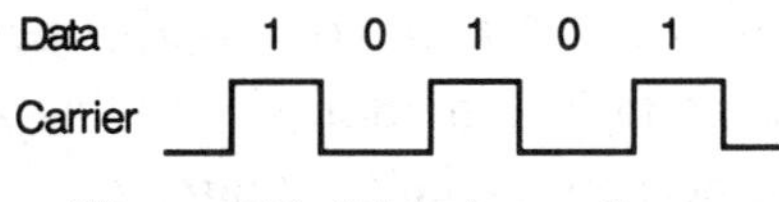

Figure 6-1 Digital encoding

Actual encoding methods are more complicated, but this method illustrates the concept.

Analog encoding imposes a continuous, sine wave data signal of a low frequency onto a carrier wave of a higher frequency. The carrier is encoded by modifying its amplitude (*amplitude modulation or AM*) or frequency (*frequency modulation or FM*) to correspond to the frequency of the data signal. Since data for communications can be analog or digital, electronic circuits are available for converting from one to another. Using these circuits, digital signals can be transmitted by analog communication and vice versa.

6.1.2 Transmission

Carriers and media come as matched pairs. The carrier is transmitted through its own medium which has been selected for minimum loss and distortion of the carrier and its encoded data. (The method for generating the carrier and other practical considerations are also used to select the medium.) Loss of carrier strength is known as *attenuation*, and changes or loss in data due to change in the carrier's properties by the medium is called *distortion*. Attenuation and distortion are measured with a unique set of units and affect the range and capacity of a communications system.

6.1.3 Attenuation

Attenuation of a carrier is expressed in *decibels* (dB). The decibel is a logarithmic unit that is calculated using the original strength of the carrier and its attenuated strength after it passes through a medium. Equations for calculation decibels vary with the unit used to express carrier strength. For example, when a carrier is light, its strength is expressed in watts. The number of decibels is calculated as

$$1 \text{ db} = 10 \log (P_1 / P_2) \qquad \text{(Equation 6.1)}$$

where

P_1 = attenuated power
P_2 = original power

Sometimes light attenuation is expressed with reference to an original power of 1 mw. This loss is called dBm and is given by

$$1 \text{ dBm} = 10 \log (P_1 / 1 \text{ mw}) \quad \text{(Equation 6.2)}$$

where

P_1 = attenuated power

6.1.4 Distortion

Distortion of the carrier can be measured by the amount of noise in the signal. *Noise* is any change in the carrier that isn't part of the encoding. The noise acts as something of a second signal in the system since it produces errant information at the receiving end, and its strength can be expressed the same way we express the strength of the carrier signal. The *signal-to-noise ratio* (SNR) is an indication of the amount of distortion in the system. The SNR can be calculated (in decibels) as

$$\text{SNR} = 10 \log (S / N) \quad \text{(Equation 6.3)}$$

where

S = the signal strength
N = the noise strength

Large values for the signal-to-noise ratio indicate the noise is much smaller than the signal, and distortion is low.

6.1.5 Capacity

The capacity of a communication system is limited by the frequency of the carrier and the bandwidth of the medium. Higher frequency carriers can carry more information, but most media impose an upper limit on frequencies above which the carrier incurs heavy attenuation. The *bandwidth of a medium* is proportional to the highest frequency the medium will transmit with a reasonable amount of attenuation. The *bandwidth of the whole communication system* indicates capacity of that system. Capacity for digital systems is expressed in the number of *bits per second* (bps) that can be transmitted. *Baud rate* is proportional to bits per second.

6.2 Fiber Optics

The advantage of light as a communications carrier lies in its extremely high frequency. Higher frequency leads to a larger capacity for data. Light offers other advantages such as immunity to electromagnetic interference, absence of electrical shock hazards, and the fact that it does not radiate out of its path (like electric signals in wire) which means the signal can't be picked up by third parties using antennae. The disadvantage of light as a carrier is that it can't be transmitted through the open air for long distances like radio, TV, or microwaves since light is absorbed and reflected by the atmosphere and since there are other sources of light that might be confused with the signal. To overcome this disadvantage, light must be contained in a medium that can be manufactured in cable form and routed from one location to another. Alternatively, it is possible to send light through areas where there is no atmosphere such as outer space.

By far the most common way to use light in communications is to pipe it through a solid rod of glass or plastic called an *optical fiber*. The fiber has an extremely small diameter (around 100 microns) and is flexible like wire.

6.2.1 How an Optical Fiber Works

As shown in Figure 6-2, light traveling from a medium with a higher index of refraction (n_1) to a medium with a lower index (n_2) will be reflected if the angle of incidence is large enough. This effect is known as *total internal reflection* and is discussed in Chapter 3.

Total internal reflection is the basis for optical fibers. The fiber is constructed of a center glass or plastic rod called the *core*. Wrapped around the core is another layer of glass or plastic called the *cladding*. The index of refraction of the core is higher than that of the cladding, and light injected into the core at the correct angle will bounce off the cladding and back into the core by total internal reflection.

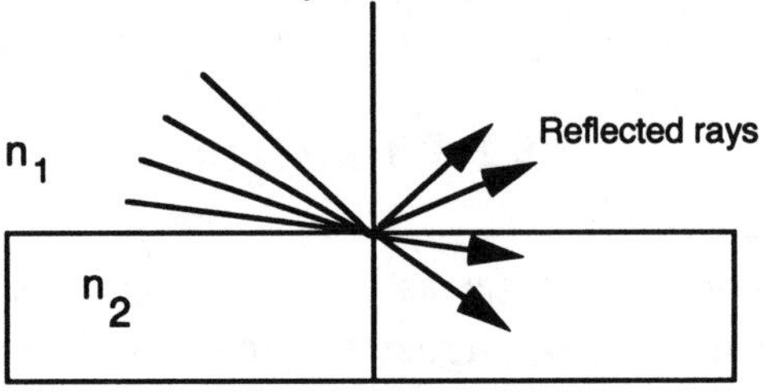

Figure 6-2 Total internal reflection
$n_1 > n_2$

As shown in Figure 6-3, light traveling through the fiber is contained through these reflections. Although both glass and plastic will work, communications grade optical fiber is made of glass because of its superior optical characteristics.

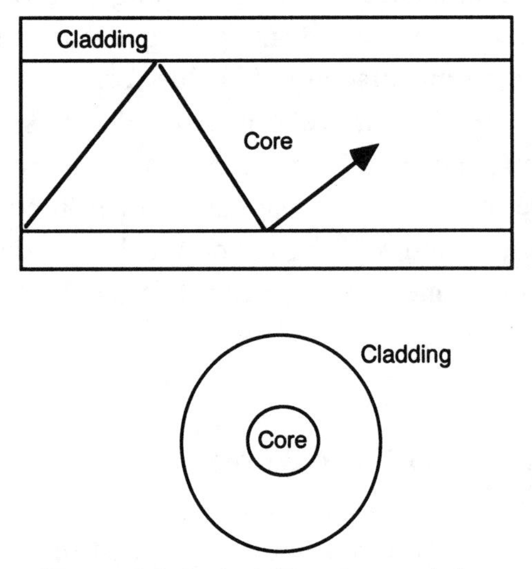

Figure 6-3 Optical fiber characteristics

6.2.2 Types of Fiber

The major types of fiber are *single mode* and *multimode*. The *modes* of a fiber can be simply defined as pathways the light follows as it travels through the core. Multimode fiber has several different pathways or modes due to the large size of its core. Light in multimode fiber will spread to fill all of these modes as it travels down the core. Since each pathway has a slightly different length, light traveling in different modes arrives at the end of the fiber at different times. This effect is called *modal dispersion* and leads to distortion.

One solution to modal dispersion is to construct a fiber so that the index of refraction of the core changes gradually from a high value in the center to a lower value near the cladding. The light traveling through this *graded index* fiber follows curved paths that are closer to the same length than in conventional *step index fiber.*

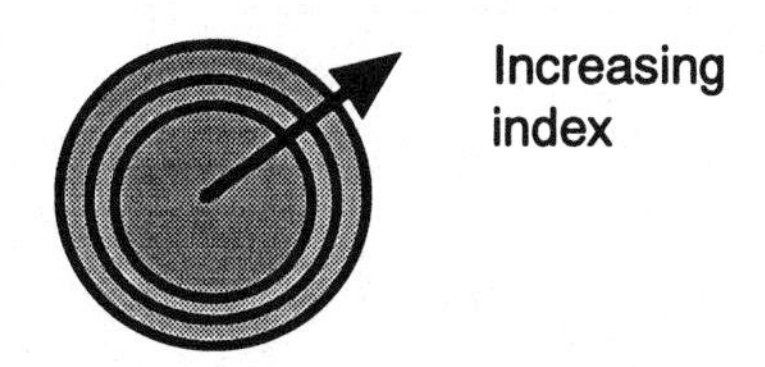

Figure 6-4 Graded index fiber

Graded index fiber reduces modal dispersion but does not eliminate it. To eliminate modal dispersion, we turn to single mode fiber. The core of a single mode fiber is made so small that there is only one mode. (The cladding is thicker so that the overall dimensions of the fiber are the same as multimode.) Because the core of single mode fiber is so small, injecting light into it becomes a much more difficult task. The light has to be collimated and focused to a small size. In this case, because of their small beam diameter and divergence, semiconductor lasers are generally preferred over ordinary light emitting diodes.

6.2.3 Attenuation and Distortion in Optical Fibers

The signal carried by light in an optical fiber is both attenuated and distorted. Attenuation is caused by absorption and scattering, and distortion results from material dispersion, modal dispersion, and waveguide effects. The distortion and attenuation can be reduced or eliminated by fiber construction, selection of light sources, and purity of fiber materials.

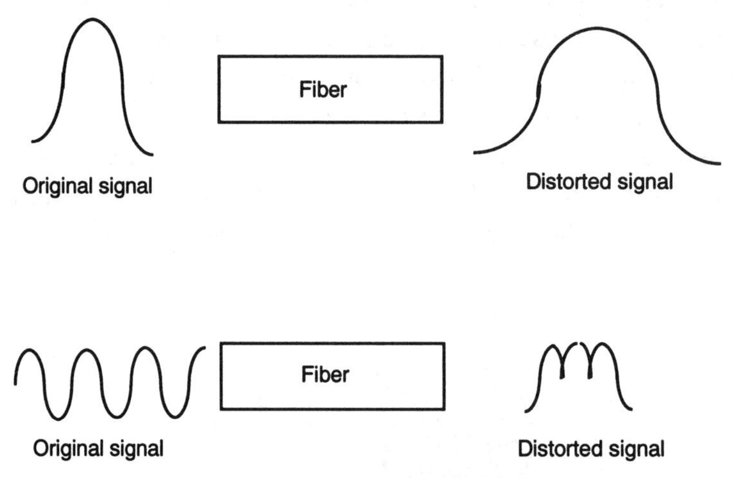

Figure 6-5 Effects of modal dispersion

Material dispersion occurs when the light passing through the fiber is made up of more than one wavelength. Since different wavelengths travel at different speeds, multiple wavelength light signals arrive at the end of the fiber with their pulses "stretched out." Figure 6-5 shows a pulse as it enters a fiber and the same pulse after the effects of material dispersion. Notice that, if several pulses were sent in a row, dispersion would cause them to overlap.

Material dispersion can be reduced by using a light source that is very closely monochromatic (such as a semiconductor laser), but since even a laser is not purely monochromatic, some material dispersion is still evident. To reduce material dispersion even further, light sources for fiber optics are generally built to emit infrared light centered around 1300 nm. The difference in speeds among the wavelengths is smallest at this point on the spectrum, and 1300 nm is sometimes called the "zero dispersion wavelength."

As mentioned in the previous sections, *modal dispersion* is caused by multiple pathways in the fiber. Since each pathway or mode is a different length, modal dispersion has the same effect as material dispersion (light arriving stretched out). Modal dispersion can be reduced with graded index fiber, or eliminated with single mode fiber. However, single mode fiber suffers from another type of dispersion known as waveguide dispersion.

Waveguide dispersion is caused by light traveling through the cladding of a single mode fiber rather than the core. Since the cladding has a different index of refraction, the light in it reaches the end of the fiber at a different time than the light in the core.

Attenuation in optical fiber is caused by scattering and absorption. Impurities in the fiber (especially water) will absorb some of the light. The amount of light absorbed depends on wavelength and generally declines as wavelength increases. There are high absorption peaks at 730 nm, 950 nm, 1250 nm, and 1380 nm due to the various types of impurities in the fiber. Fortunately, absorption is relatively low at the zero dispersion wavelength of 1300 nm. Some specialized fibers, known as *dispersion shifted,* are designed so that zero dispersion wavelength is shifted to 1550 nm to take advantage of its lower absorption.

Scattering is caused by impurities and imperfections (such as cracks and bubbles) and also causes attenuation. There are different types of scattering, but the dominant type in optical fiber is Raleigh scattering. Raleigh scattering losses are inversely proportional to the wavelength of light raised to the fourth power. Longer wavelengths (like 1300 nm and 1550 nm) scatter less.

6.2.4 Fiber-Optic Transmitters and Receivers

Fiber-optic transmitters are equipped with either *light-emitting diodes* (LED's) or *semiconductor lasers*. The LED is much less expensive, but it emits light with a broader range of wavelengths and in a wider beam than a laser. LED's also emit much less power. For short and medium distance applications, the cost advantage of LED's outweighs its disadvantages. The losses incurred in short distances and the distortion due to different wavelengths is small in short distances; and the fiber used (multimode) has a larger numerical aperture.

Numerical aperture (NA) is an indication of how narrow a beam of light must be to enter the core of a fiber. A fiber's numerical aperture is defined in terms of its cone of acceptance or physical limits that the beam must fit, as shown in Figure 6-6. Numerical aperture is the sine of the angle of the cone of acceptance.

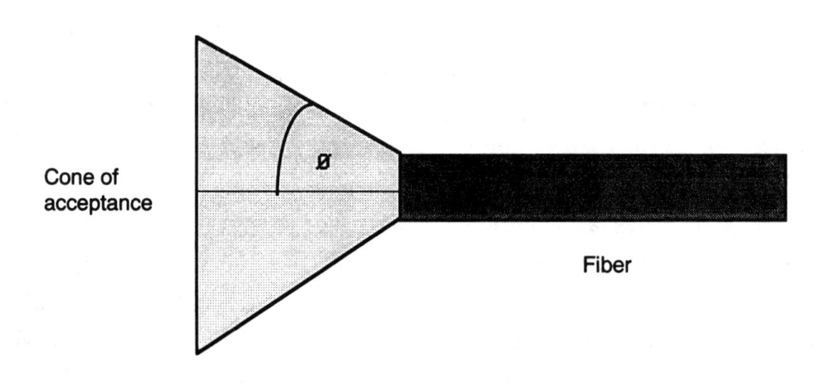

Figure 6-6 Numerical aperture
N.A. = sine Ø

Since multimode fiber has a large N.A., LED's are a viable light source. Longer distance fiber applications use single mode fiber to reduce distortion and semiconductor lasers because of their higher power and smaller beam diameter. Both lasers and LED's are modulated by modulating the current of their power supply.

Fiber-optic receivers detect light with photosensitive semiconductor devices. The *PIN photodiode* offers a low-cost detector that detects light through the *photoconductive* effect. Light incident on a reverse biased PIN photodiode causes an increase in current proportional to the amount of light. *Avalanche photodiodes* (APD) are much more sensitive devices that provide high current outputs for small amounts of incident light. APD's are much more expensive and require a fairly high bias voltage (on the order of 100 v). Choice of detector—much like choice of light source—depends on the distance involved, cost, and the amount of light received at the end of the fiber.

6.2.5 Fiber-Optic Connectors and Splices

Joining two fibers together, whether permanently as in splices or temporarily as in connectors, is a difficult task. The cores of fibers must be aligned and the ends of the fiber must touch so that light can travel through the joint uninterrupted. Aligning the fibers using their claddings can cause trouble if the cores are not precisely centered or not exactly round. To make sure the fibers butt up evenly, the ends are generally polished so they are flat and even. Burrs or gouges in the end of the fiber would leave air gaps that would cause the light to reflect at the joint and be lost.

To connect two fibers, each end is placed in a precision manufactured plastic (or sometimes metal) sleeve that has a means of holding the fiber in place. The two sleeves then join together through tabs and notches or by threads. Many fiber connectors are built so that they are similar to standard copper wire connectors. *SMA, SMC, and SMB* connectors are examples of these. Some connectors, like the *dry no polish* (DNP) type, are meant for low-cost applications where loss in the connection is not critical.

Fiber-optic splices can take advantage of the fact that the join is permanent and not to be undone. The *elastomeric* splice holds the fiber ends in place with channels cut into a rubber-like material that is placed into two halves of a cylinder cut lengthwise. Often an *index matching gel* is injected in the splice to fill any gaps between the fiber and reduce loss. Other *mechanical* splices use similar clamps or holders to keep the two fibers in position.

Fusion splicing is the most effective way of splicing fibers together. A fusion splicer melts the ends of the fiber together with an electric arc. The ends of the fiber are aligned with micropositioning stages that are operated manually or are automatically controlled with an electronic circuit that makes adjustments based on light passing through the joint. Some models even provide a camera that displays the splicing process on a television screen and extra circuitry to calculate the loss caused by the splice. However, fusion splicers are expensive and require some specialized training to operate.

6.3 Optical Storage Devices

With the rapid growth of computer systems, storage of large volumes of data has become an important field. As with most areas of electronics, the push is toward larger and larger capacity in a smaller space. Consumer electronics for entertainment, such as audio and video products, has also created a storage demand. This time quality and lifetime are the important parameters.

Optical storage devices have been created to match these demands. As with most types of storage, optical storage involves modifying the properties of a storage medium to represent information. Retrieving data from the medium is known as *reading*, while recording data is called *writing*. Devices that do not allow the user to record data are referred to as *read only* devices.

By far the most common optical storage medium is a compact disk, but new, erasable, technologies are becoming more viable.

6.3.1 Compact Disks

Compact disks (CD's) are thin disks made of polycarbonate capable of storing large amounts of data in a digital format. The CD is read by scanning it with the beam of a semiconductor laser. Since the laser has no physical contact with the disk, there is no wear from repeated use.

The compact disk is a thin, circular piece of polycarbonate with a hole in the center. The disk is 12 cm in diameter, and information is molded into the disk in the form of *pits* and *lands* that represent binary numbers (see Figure 6-7). The pits are 0.12 microns deep and 0.6 microns wide. Lands vary in size from 0.9 to 3.3 microns. The lands and pits are in a spiral pattern from the center of the disk outward, and each spiral is separated by about 1.6 microns. After molding, the disk is coated with a reflective layer of aluminum and then with a transparent protective layer.

Information is read from a disk by a laser beam. The laser beam scans the underside of the disk from the center outward radially while the disk rotates (see Figure 6-8). The beam is passed through a polarizing beam splitter (PBS) before it reaches the disk, and the reflected beam also passes through the PBS. The incident and reflected beams interfere at a detector that measures the intensity of the light. Light intensity from a land reflection will be different than that from a pit reflection due to the difference in phase shift and the resulting interference effects (see Chapter 3).

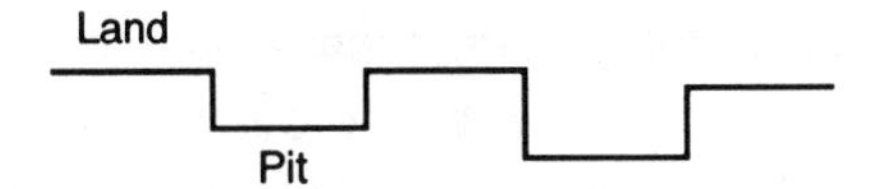

Figure 6-7 Surface of a CD

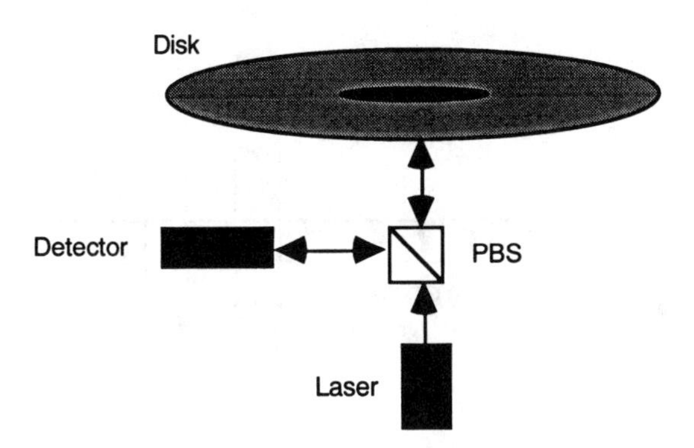

Figure 6-8 Reading a CD

Because the information stored on the CD can't be changed by the user, CD's are read only mediums. CD readers for computers are often known as *WORM* drives (for Write Once Read Many), and the CD's themselves are called *CD-ROM* where ROM stands fore Read Only Memory. In the entertainment market, CD's are used to store audio data which can be retrieved with a CD player connected to a stereo system. *Laser Video Disks* (LVD), a related technology, are used for storing movies and other video information. Audio, video, and computer data on CD devices have found a niche in education as part of multimedia presentation equipment. Laser video is also used along with a host computer for interactive tutorials that provide the user with video and audio information and accept input (in the form of answers to questions, etc.) via the computer keyboard.

6.3.2 Erasable Optical Disks

The major drawback of compact disks is that they are not erasable. Several new optical storage technologies have been created to address that problem. These new technologies combine the advantages of no contact and high storage density with a storage material that can be erased and written on with the same unit that reads the data. The two most developed erasable optical storage technologies are magneto-optic and phase change.

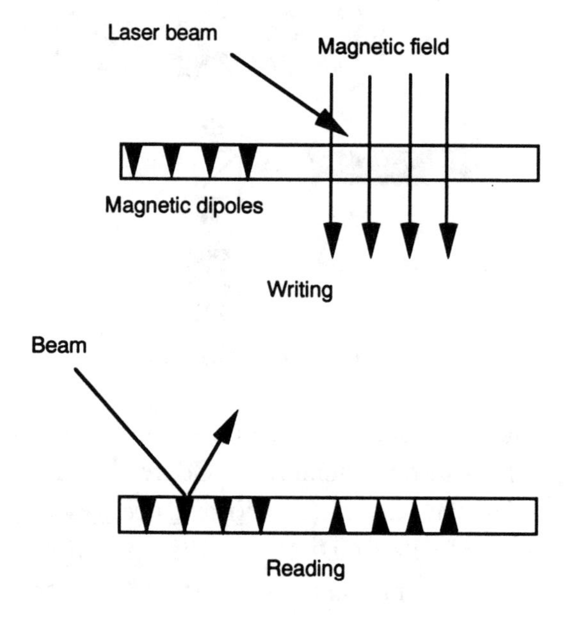

Figure 6-9 Magneto-optic storage

Magneto-optic uses a storage method similar to the magnetic storage of floppy disk systems. The storage medium contains millions of magnetic dipoles, each representing bits of digital data. As shown in

Figure 6-9, each magnetic dipole represents information by its orientation (for example, north pole up for a "1" and down for a "0"). To write data, an electric field is applied to an area of the media along with a laser beam that increases its temperature. Since the medium (usually terbium and iron) is more susceptible to changes in magnetic field orientation at higher temperatures, the laser beam is used to cause the changes that would not normally occur at room temperature.

A lower powered laser beam is scanned across the magneto-optic material to read it. The polarization of the reflected beam will be altered differently depending on the orientation of the magnetic field it strikes.

Phase change recording in optical storage is accomplished using a medium that can be changed from a highly reflective crystalline state to a low reflective amorphous state. State changes are caused by the interaction between a higher power beam and the material. Reading is accomplished using a lower beam. Phase change disks are made of tellurium suboxide alloyed with germanium, lead, and indium.

6.4 Information Manipulation

Information can be retrieved, transferred, or combined using optical technology. The major areas in information manipulation by lasers are barcode scanning and laser printing. Both applications take advantage of the directability of the laser beam.

6.4.1 Barcodes

Barcodes are labels made up of a series of dark lines separated by white spaces. These labels are codes for numbers and letters and are read by scanning light. A detector is used to pick up the light reflected from the label; the amount of light reflected and the duration of the reflections are used to interpret the data stored on the label. Barcode labels are used extensively in retail stores (especially grocery) where the merchandise is labeled, and the cash register is equipped with a counter laser scanner like the one shown in Figure 6-10, or a handheld scanner. The cash register reads the label via the scanner and uses the information to recall price and update inventory records.

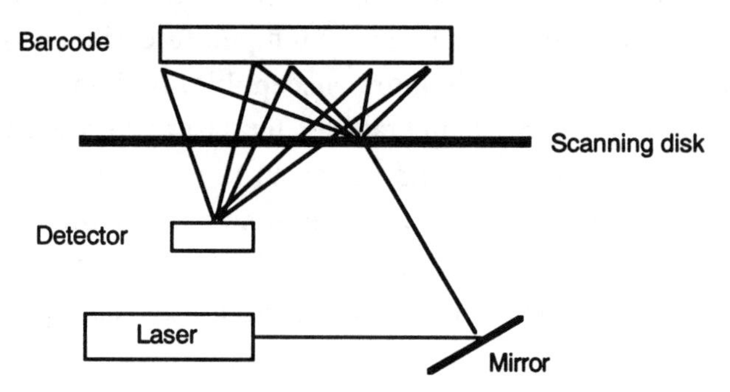

Figure 6-10 Barcode scanner

6.4.2 Laser Printers

Laser printers are used to produce high-quality documents with a personal computer system. Figure 6-11 shows a typical laser printer setup. A laser beam is passed through an acousto-optic modulator which pulses the beam before it reflects from a rotating mirror and is scanned onto a photosensitive cylinder.

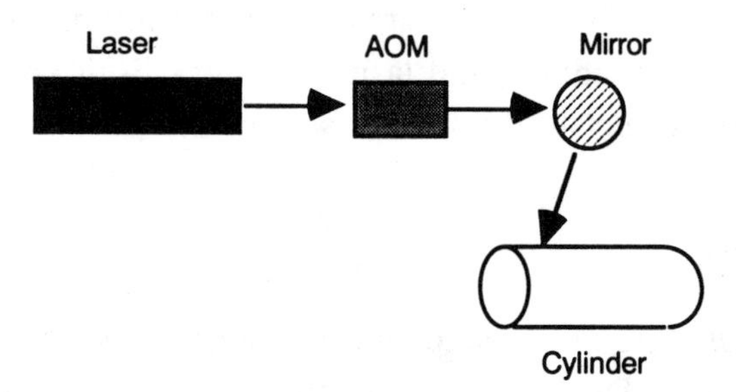

Figure 6-11 Schematic diagram for a laser printer

The surface of the cylinder is initially covered with a positive charge that will be removed when irradiated by the laser beam. A negatively charged ink (or toner) is brushed onto the cylinder which is then rolled onto a positively charged sheet of paper. The toner sticks to the paper and forms an image. In addition to high-quality text, some laser printers are also capable of producing high-quality graphics and several sizes and styles of fonts.

BIBLIOGRAPHY

"CD ROM's: The Laser's Edge in Data Storage" *Mechanical Engineering*. April, 1987.

Desmarais, Norman. "Laser Libraries" *Byte* May, 1986.

Hecht, Jeff. "Lasers Store a Wealth of Data" *High Technology*. May/June, 1982.

Rothchild, Edward. "Optical Memory: Data Storage by Laser" *Byte*. October, 1984.

Sterling, Donald J. *A Technician's Guide to Fiber Optics* Albany: Delmar Publishers, 1987.

7

MEDICAL APPLICATIONS

Introduction

The properties of a laser that make it effective in materials processing (its concentrated energy) are also the reason the laser plays an increasingly larger role in therapeutic medical applications. The intense energy provided by medium- and high-powered lasers allows surgeons to cut tissue and cauterize the incision at the same time, prompting the laser's nickname, "the bloodless scalpel." Since various wavelengths of light are absorbed at different levels by different types of tissue, the laser is also a highly selective scalpel. The surface area and depth of the laser beam's effects can be precisely controlled by taking advantage of these special tissue properties and by controlling the beam parameters. Several lasers play roles in medicine, but the Nd:YAG and the CO_2 are the main surgical lasers. Argon lasers are used in some opthamological applications and the excimer laser has shown some unique advantages in special areas of treatment.

The areas of medicine that take advantage of laser surgery are varied and growing in number, but primarily the laser can be found in ophthalmology, dermatology, and some forms of surgery on internal organs. To explain the role of the laser in medicine, this chapter focuses on the unique absorption properties of tissues in the human body. The effects of the beam when it is absorbed are then discussed, and, finally, some common applications are described in detail.

7.1 Light Absorption by Tissue and Other Organic Material

7.1.1 Wavelength Dependence

The basis for any laser beam effect lies in the amount of light the target material will absorb. In tissue, as with other materials, this absorption is wavelength dependent. Absorption of visible and near infrared wavelengths depends on the amount and type of *pigment* in the tissue. Pigment is the chemical in tissues that gives them color. Some important pigments are melanin in the skin and hemoglobin in blood cells. Larger amounts of melanin cause dark tissue, while smaller amounts are found in light tissue. Hemoglobin lends a red color to red blood cells. Darker color from melanin means more absorption throughout the visible spectrum and into near infrared, but hemoglobin, because of its red color, absorbs highly at the green end of the spectrum but reflects red and near infrared light.

In the far infrared (greater than about 2 μm), tissue absorption loses its wavelength dependence and remains constant regardless of wavelength. Ultraviolet light is the least studied range for tissue absorption, primarily because easily available UV laser light is a relatively new phenomena.

7.1.2 Depth of Penetration

The depth of penetration of the laser beam also depends on wavelength. Some tissues have a high *absorption coefficient* which means they absorb most of the incident light before it can penetrate too deeply. Tissues with low absorption coefficients allow light to pass through to a greater depth. The absorption coefficient of tissue depends on the wavelength of the laser beam throughout most of the visible and near infrared spectrum, but is constant in the far infrared. At the longer far infrared wavelengths, the beam penetration is limited to the surface of the tissue.

Depth of penetration can be calculated for a tissue/wavelength combination with a known absorption coefficient. Since the beam does not abruptly stop at a given depth but gradually loses power as it penetrates, penetration depth is defined as the point where the laser beam is reduced to half its original intensity. *Penetration depth* ($X_{1/2}$) is given by:

$$X_{1/2} = (1/a)\ln 2 \qquad \text{(Equation 7.1)}$$

where

a = absorption coefficient.

Figure 7-1 illustrates the typical penetration depth for various wavelengths. Notice penetration is high in the visible region of the spectrum (under 2,000 nm) and tapers off substantially in the far infrared.

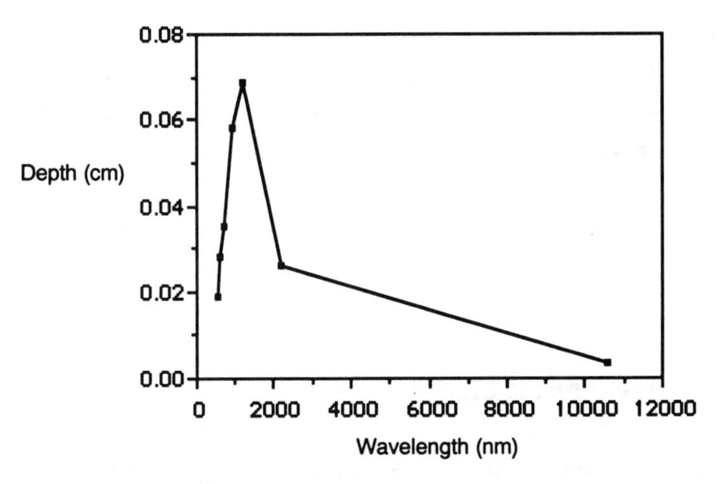

Figure 7-1 Penetration depth vs. wavelength

When calculating penetration depth and the effects of absorption, the cooling effects of circulating blood and the thermal diffusivity of the tissue need to be considered. As the beam heats the tissue, the blood circulating around the area of interaction will remove some of the heat. Recall from Chapter 5 that heat flows away from the beam through the rest of the material as well. The amount of heat lost by this flow is governed by the tissue's thermal diffusivity. Taking these effects into consideration, the *net temperature change of the tissue* (ΔT) is given by:

$$\Delta T = (E_{net}\ a)/[2(\ln a)Cp] \qquad \text{(Equation 7.2)}$$

where

E_{net} = energy absorbed
C = specific heat, and
p = density.

The specific heat of tissue is approximately 3.6 j/g°C and the density is approximately 1.2 g/cm^3.

7.2 Effects of Light Absorption of Tissue

Light absorption effects on tissue are divided into two categories. *Photochemical effects* are chemical changes (usually breaking of molecular bonds) caused by the light. Photoablation and photodynamic therapy are two examples. *Thermal effects* are the result of the tissue increasing in temperature after absorbing the light. Two thermal effects are photocoagulation and photovaporization. Thermal effects vary in proportion to the amount of temperature change.

7.2.1 Photochemical Effects

Photoablation. Photoablation is the technical term for removing tissue cells by breaking their molecular bonds. Since a cell is composed of several molecules bonded together, energy from a laser beam can be used to remove the cell by breaking the bonds. The cell is broken up by the incoming beam.

The uses of photoablation are similar to photovaporization since they both generally result in an incision or excision. However, the term photoablation is used to identify the effect of ultraviolet beams from excimer lasers, while photovaporization generally results from an infrared beam.

Photodynamic therapy. Photodynamic therapy involves introducing a light sensitive chemical (hematoporphyrin) into a specific group of cells (usually intravenously). The cells are then subjected to light from a laser and the photosensitive chemical reacts and destroys the cells. This process allows selective removal of cells in a very controlled manner. As shown in Figure 7-2, the incoming beam would effect only the treated cells (black circles) while the untreated cells (white circles) would not react.

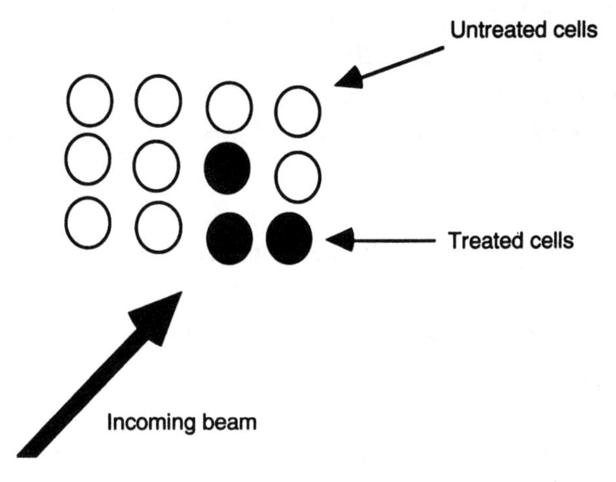

Figure 7-2 Photodynamic therapy

7.2.2 Thermal Effects

Photovaporization. Photovaporization removes cells by heating the cell and surrounding material (solid and liquid) to the point where they change into a gas. Since water composes the largest part of this material, heating a cell to the boiling point of water (100°C) causes vaporization. Equation 7.2 in the previous section can be used to determine the amount of beam power required to vaporize cells.

When photovaporization is used in surgery, the resulting incision will not bleed because the cells neighboring the incision are sealed off by the heat of the beam. This effect is known as cauterizing.

Photocoagulation. Photocoagulation is caused by heating the cells to a high enough temperature (70°C) to kill them. The dead cells then form scar tissue which can be used to bridge between different areas of tissue (for example, reattaching torn muscles). The clotting of the scar tissue also stops blood flow. Normal body temperature of tissue is 37°C, so temperature changes of 63°C for durations of one second or longer will kill cells and form scar tissue. Applying Equation 7.2 to fair skin irradiated with a Nd:YAG laser beam (with an absorption coefficient of 10.1 cm^{-1}), a temperature change of 63°C requires a net energy of 37.4 joules, Since fair skin reflects about 60% of the Nd:YAG beam, the laser would actually need to provide about 62 $joules/cm^2$ (40% above the required amount) for one second or longer to cause photocoagulation.

7.3 Lasers in Ophthalmology

7.3.1 Basic Parts of the Eye

The eye is an excellent candidate for therapeutic laser applications because it is constructed specifically for capturing and focusing light. The basic structure of the eye is shown in Figure 7-3. Light enters the eye through the *pupil* and is focused by the *lens* onto the *retina*. The retina converts the light to electrical pulses which are sent down the *optic nerve* to the brain. The *iris* widens or contracts to control the amount of light entering the eye. The *cornea* provides a protective shell for the eye.

Because the eye "sees" visible light, light in the visible and near infrared portions of the spectrum passes through the cornea, the pupil, and the lens and is focused on the retina. Far infrared and ultraviolet light are absorbed by the cornea. For this reason, retinal work is usually done with visible light lasers like the argon and the ruby or near infrared lasers like the Nd:YAG. Cornea work requires the far infrared beam of a CO_2 or the ultraviolet beam of an excimer laser.

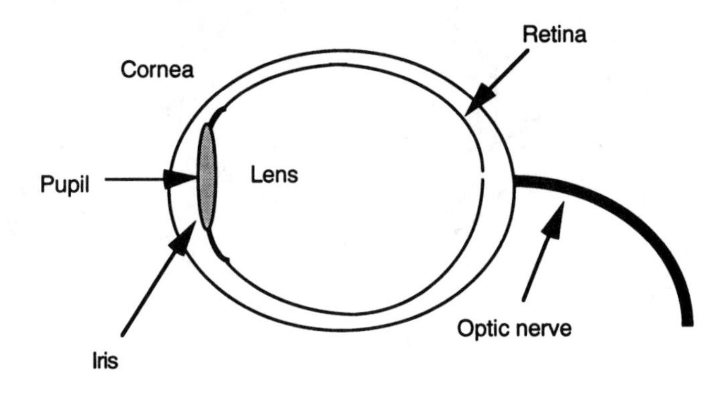

Figure 7-3 Basic parts of the eye

7.3.2 Example—Retinal Detachment

One major type of laser eye surgery involves curing *retinal detachment*. The retina can be detached from its underlying tissue due to inflammation, splitting of retinal layers, or small holes in the retina. The retina is reattached by exposing it to the focused beam from a ruby or argon laser. The beam passes through the front of the eye and is focused by the lens of the eye onto different areas of the retina.

The beam causes photocoagulation which forms scar tissue that bridges the gap between the retina and the tissue behind. The laser offers the advantage of allowing reattachment at specific points without damaging the surrounding area of the retina. A pulsed beam with a short duration will accomplish the reattachment in a very short time span so that the patient doesn't have a chance to move. The photocoagulation is controlled by adjusting the power or energy of the beam, and the beam may be delivered to the eye through an optical fiber.

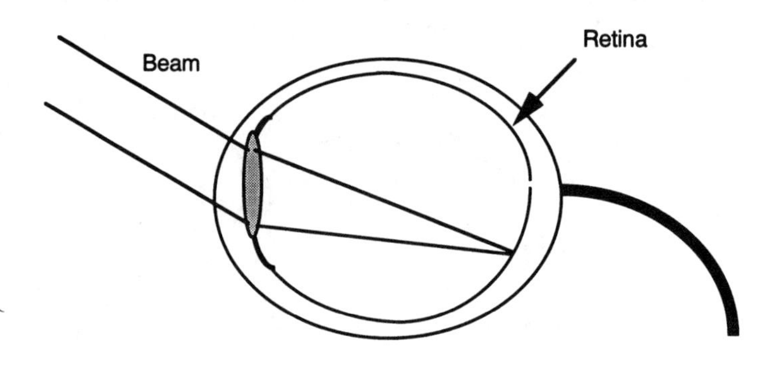

Figure 7-4 Retinal detachment surgery

7.3.3 Example—Diabetic Retinopathy

Diabetic retinopathy, another eye disorder, occurs in the eyes of people with diabetes. Abnormal blood vessels form in the retina and may hemorrhage (bleed). The bleeding destroys surrounding tissues and can lead to blindness. The abnormal blood vessels contain hemoglobin which absorbs the green beam from an argon laser. The argon beam is used to seal off the vessels by photocoagulation before they hemorrhage.

Resculpting the cornea with a laser beam to correct vision defects is currently in the experimental stage. The beam from an argon fluoride laser is used to change the profile of the cornea, and the front surface of the cornea (epithelium) regenerates about two days after the operation. The laser beam is not as risky as a diamond knife or radial keratotomy (two technologies that are currently used).

7.4 Lasers in Dermatology

The absorption properties of skin tissue provide an opportunity for laser applications in removal of skin blemishes. The laser beam has been used to remove the "port wine stain" birthmark and tattoos. The beam of an argon laser applied to these areas of the skin causes lightening of the skin, and since surrounding, unblemished skin is not as absorbent, the beam only affects the tattoo or stain.

Lasers have also been used to remove warts or tumors by photovaporization. The beam causes incision and simultaneous cauterization which removes the growth without bleeding. Common types of growths that have been removed by lasers include vascular lesions, keloids, and hyperplastic lesions.

7.5 Diagnostic Applications

In addition to the therapeutic applications mentioned above, the laser lends itself to some unique diagnostic procedures. By scanning areas with a laser beam, physicians can determine their size, shape, and velocity. Because of the unique structure of the eye, diagnostic laser applications are most prominent in ophthalmology.

The resolving power of the retina can be found using a type of interferometry (see Chapter 8). High contrast interference patterns are produced in the patient's eye, and the patient identifies the smallest fringe separation he or she can distinguish. This test gives a measurement of the acuity of the retina.

The reflections of a laser beam scanned across the retina can be collected and used to create a video image of the retina. A more focused beam can be used to measure the speed of blood vessels flowing in the retina via velocimetry. A laser beam can also be used to stimulate parts of a retina—the resulting response provides a map of the sensitivity of the retina and indicates abnormalities.

BIBLIOGRAPHY

Council on Scientific Affairs "Lasers in Medicine and Surgery" *Journal of the American Medical Association.* vol. 256, no. 7, August 15, 1986.

Course VIII, Laser Applications Waco, Texas: CORD, 1980.

Hecht, Jeff, "Lasers to Find New Uses in Medical and Dental Treatment" *Lasers & Optronics,* June, 1989.

8

LASERS IN ANALYSIS AND TESTING

Introduction

Distance measurement, non-destructive testing, spectroscopy, or other forms of analysis and testing are fields where the laser is used extensively. The laser beam's coherence allows the use of interference effects to discover changes in stressed objects and minute changes in distance, while the directionality of the beam provides for long-distance projection and rangefinding. Monochromatic laser light is useful in studying the absorption and fluorescence of a wide range of materials. Chapter 8 covers the fundamentals of interferometry, and its applications in testing. Rangefinding methods, spectroscopy, and fiber-optic sensors are discussed as well.

8.1 Interferometry

Coherent laser light has a fixed phase relationship. If the laser beam is divided into two parts and a phase shift is introduced, then the recombined beam will show interference patterns. Light that has a zero degree's phase shift will *constructively interfere* to form a bright fringe;, while light that is out of phase will *destructively interfere* to form a dark fringe. (The principles of interference were discussed in detail in Chapter 3.)

8.1.1 Standard Interferometers

Michelson's Interferometer. Interference effects are illustrated in a device known as a *Michelson interferometer*. As shown in Figure 8-1, the interferometer divides the light from a coherent source (in this case a laser) into two parts.

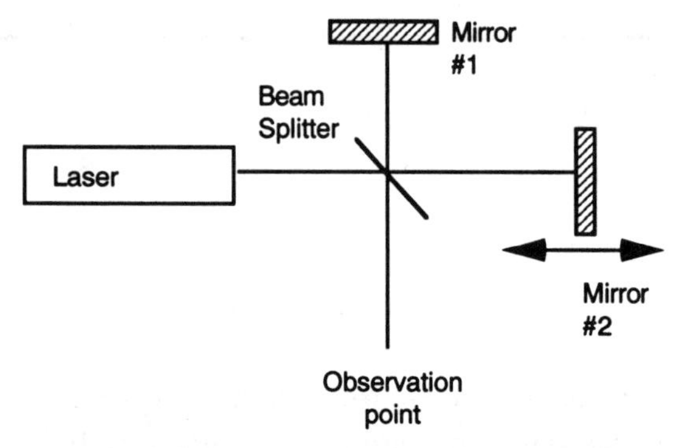

Figure 8-1 Michelson's interferometer

Part A travels from the beam splitter to mirror #1 and then back through the beam splitter to the observation point. Part B travels from the beam splitter to mirror #2 and then back to the observation point. At the observation point the two parts recombine to form interference patterns. The light that is *in phase* will form bright fringes, while the light that is *out of phase* will form dark rings. A precisely aligned system (both mirrors are straight and perpendicular to one another) will produce a pattern like that shown in Figure 8-2.

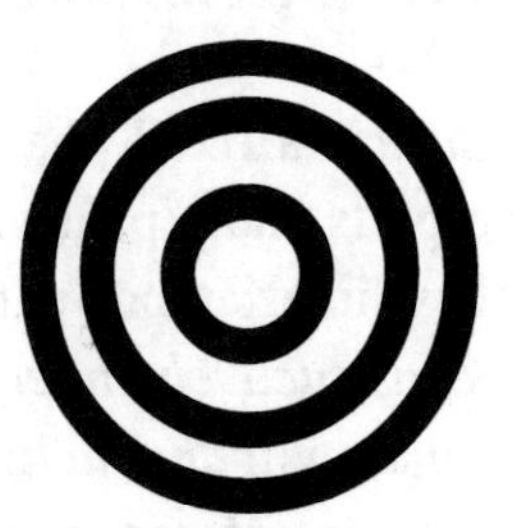

Figure 8-2 Interference pattern

Applications of Michelson's Interferometer. Michelson's interferometer can be used to measure small changes in the position of mirror #2. If the mirror (which is moveable) is translated toward or away from the beam splitter, the rings in the interference pattern will expand away from or collapse toward the center, due to changes in phase caused by the change in distance. By counting the number of rings (m) that move past an arbitrary point, the distance that mirror #2 is moved (d) is calculated as shown in Equation 8.1:

$$d = m\,\lambda \qquad \text{(Equation 8.1)}$$

where λ is the wavelength of light used. For practical distance measurements, mirror #2 of the interferometer would be mounted on an object whose distance was to be measured.

Index of refraction measurements can be made with the interferometer as well. A material placed in one leg of the interferometer will cause a phase shift because its index of refraction is different from the air in the other leg. This phase shift, like the movement of a mirror, will cause the rings in the interference pattern to move.

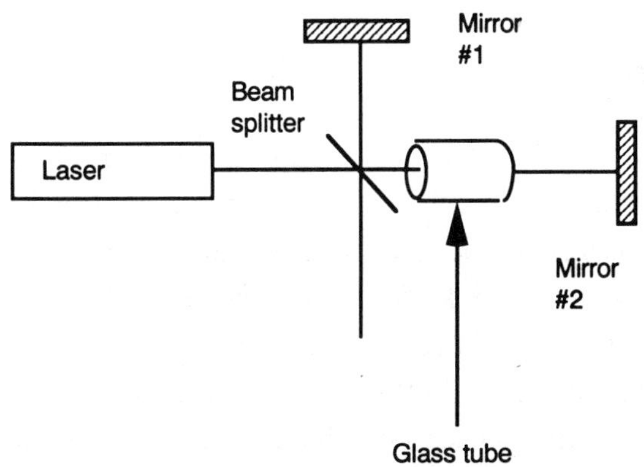

Figure 8-3 Index of refraction measurement

Figure 8-3 is a diagram of the setup used to measure the index of refraction of a gas. The glass tube is evacuated and the gas is allowed to fill the tube slowly. As gas fills the tube, the shift in interference fringes is observed. The index of refraction (n) of the gas can be calculated by using the number of fringes (m), the wavelength of the light (λ), and the length of the tube (t) in the following formula:

$$n = 1 + (m\lambda)/t \quad \text{(Equation 8.2)}$$

Other Standard Interferometers. Although Michelson's interferometer is a common example, there are many other interferometer designs. All of them are based on the same principle as Michelson's, but they make use of different optical arrangements and have different applications. The table below summarizes some other interferometers.

Table 8-1 Interferometer Summary

Interferometer	Application
Twyman-Green	Testing optical components -- lenses and flats.
Mach-Zender	Measuring flow patterns in wind tunnels.
Jamin	Measuring indexes of refraction.

8.1.2 Holographic Interferometry

Principles of Holography. *Holograms* are true three-dimensional pictures formed by the interference effects of a laser beam. To understand holography, it helps to take a look at normal photography. A photograph is an image formed on a piece of film or a glass plate by capturing light reflected from an object. Figure 8-4 shows a functional diagram of the process. Light reflected from an object is gathered and focused by a set of optics. The photographic film records the image by recording the intensity of light reflected by each point on the object. The light causes a chemical reaction in the film that results in dark areas on the film. The aggregate of these dark areas forms a two-dimensional image of the object.

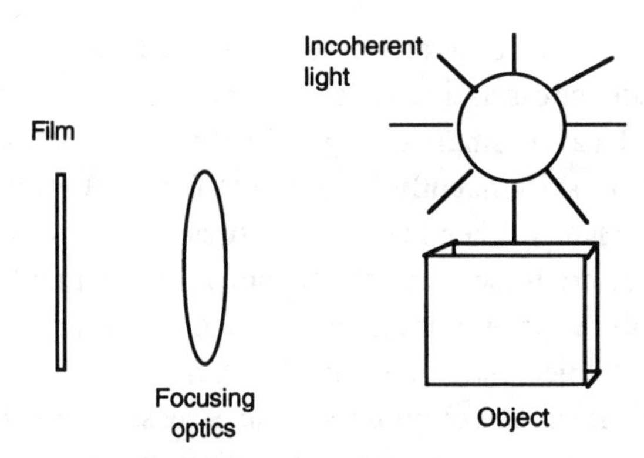

Figure 8-4 Normal photography

The photograph is two-dimensional because it represents an image of the reflectivity (or shades) of the object. It does not provide information about the location of each part of the object relative to another part. In order to include this information, a process for recording the depth of the object is required.

Holography records the depth of the object by interference effects. Figure 8-5 shows the setup for a transmission hologram. The light that reflects off the object (object beam) interferes with the light in the reference beam. The resulting patterns are a function of the difference in distance traveled by the two beams. Since the object beam must travel longer (or shorter) distances to reach various points on the object, the interference effects of the film are a recording of the depth of the object.

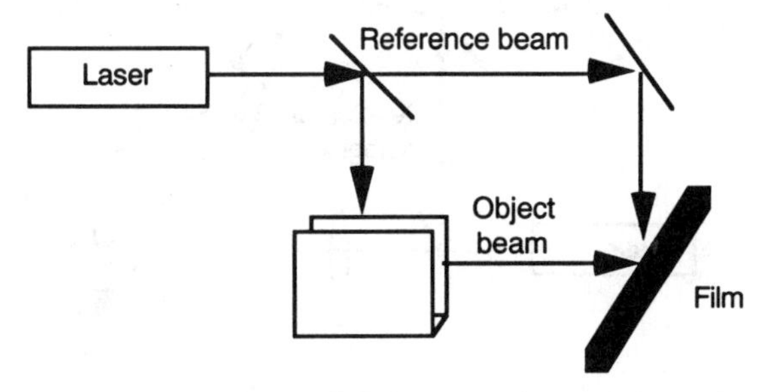

Figure 8-5 Holography

Holographic Interferometry. Holography has several applications, but as a tool for testing it has expanded the principles of interferometry.

Holographic interferometry is used to study microscopic changes in objects under stress as a result of vibration, strain, etc. Since stress on an object will cause small changes in the object's shape, interference patterns (and subsequently holograms) formed by reflections from the object will change when the object is stressed.

There are three principal methods for holographic interferometry. The double exposure method relies on making a hologram of an undisturbed object, stressing the object, and re-exposing the same piece of film to form a hologram of the stressed object. The resulting hologram reveals the changes to the object caused by the stress. Double exposure holography uses the same procedures and equipment as any holographic process and therefore offers the advantage of simplicity. However, double exposure is limited to objects that remain motionless once they are stressed.

Real time holography (Figure 8-6) provides a view of the changes in the object as they occur. It is not necessary to wait for the hologram to be developed before analyzing the stress. In real time holography, a hologram is made of the object and then the image formed by the hologram is made to overlap that object. Viewing the object through the original hologram allows the experimenter to see any subsequent changes in the object due to stress as they occur.

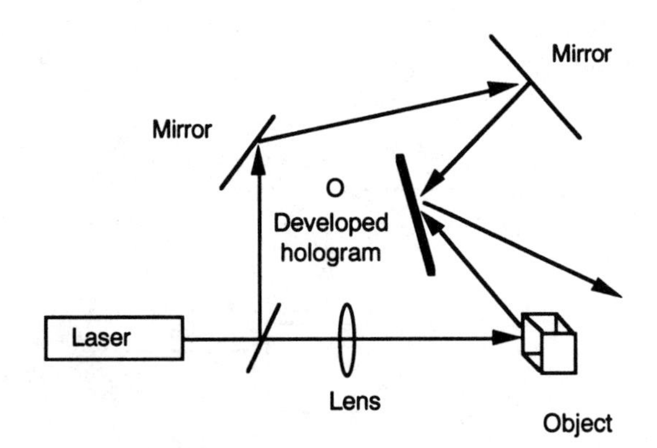

Figure 8-6 Real time holography
(Object is viewed through developed hologram at point O)

Time average holography is used when the object goes through a large number of changes in a short period of time (e.g., when the object is vibrating). A hologram is made by exposing the film for a relatively long duration. The resulting hologram will be an averaged version of the several images formed during the exposure and will reveal which parts of the object remained stationary (bright fringes in the hologram) and which parts are vibrating.

Applications of Holographic Interferometry. Holographic interferometry is used in the nondestructive testing of manufactured parts and materials. By using one of the holographic techniques discussed above, the stress a part would normally experience in use can be simulated and possible weak points can be isolated. The holographic picture of the part will indicate areas that change their physical shape by a relatively large amount as compared to other areas. Such distorted areas can be weak spots on the part and are susceptible to breaking or cracking during use.

As an example, consider a tire manufacturer trying to determine possible weak points in a tire. By using holographic interferometry, the tire without stress (no air) can be compared to the tire under stress (filled with air). The parts of the tire that show bulging or distortion in shape under pressure are possible weak points. The manufacturer can compare the information about the tire found through interferometry to set standards for the tire in order to decide whether the tire is road worthy. Information about the process used in manufacturing the tire can also be deduced from the testing information.

8.2 Rangefinding

The directivity of the laser beam combined with its unique optical properties make it a useful tool for measuring distances. The laser is used to measure distances as small as a wavelength of light and as large as several meters or even kilometers. In every case the properties of the laser beam allow for highly accurate measurements. There are several methods for measuring distance using a laser, including the interferometric techniques discussed in the previous section. This section will concentrate on methods normally used for longer distances.

In these methods, distance is determined by measuring the time it takes the laser beam to reach the target (object whose distance is to be measured) and return. Since the speed of light (v) is a known value, distance (d) is calculated by measuring the time (t) and using Equation 8.3.

$$d = v\, t \qquad \text{(Equation 8.3)}$$

The actual calculations used in laser distance measurement are more complex because the distortion of the laser beam as it passes through the atmosphere must be taken into account.

Consider the block diagram of a laser distance measurement system shown in Figure 8-7. The laser beam is collimated by a set of optics to reduce its divergence. This is done so the laser beam will not spread into an unmanageable size as it travels toward the target and then returns.

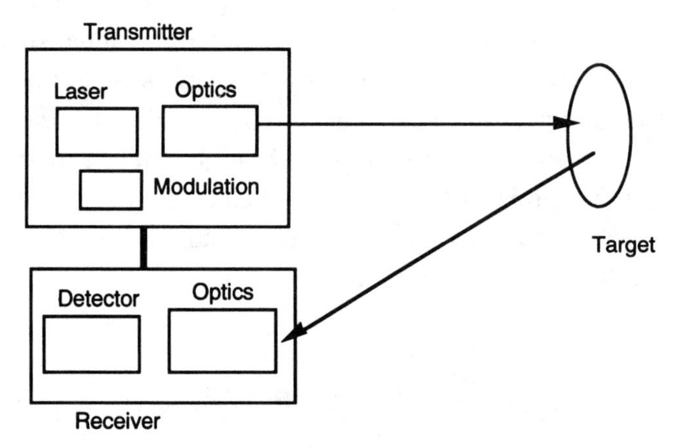

Figure 8-7 Block diagram of laser distance measurement system

The beam reflects from the target and is gathered by another set of optics at the receiver. This second set of optics is designed to gather and focus all the reflected laser light possible. Often, a filter is added to block out any light that is not part of the laser beam. As the beam travels through the space between the target and the distance measurement device, it loses power (due to absorption) and increases in diameter (due to divergence). Further changes in the beam may be caused by the target, depending on its nature. If the target is made up of a special device (usually a mirror) that has been made to enhance the reflection of the beam, and placed in position, the laser beam will experience only a minimum distortion. If the target is what is known as noncooperative (meaning it is not specially designed to reflect the beam), then the beam may lose power due to low reflectivity and may even change shape.

The effects of the optics in the transmitter and receiver and the effects of the target are incorporated into the calculations used to discover distance. The actual effects vary from system to system. They can be summed up in a few terms. The *transmitted power density* (P_{trans}) is a function of the size and nature of the transmitter optics and the power and divergence of the laser. The *power density at the target* (P_{tar}) is the transmitted power density multiplied by the loss caused by absorption by the atmosphere (T).

$$P_{tar} = P_{trans} * T \qquad \text{(Equation 8.4)}$$

The *power density reflected from the target* (P_{ref}) is the power density at the target times the reflectivity of the target and a factor used to express the size of the target (D_{tar}).

$$P_{ref} = P_{tar} * D_{tar} \qquad \text{(Equation 8.5)}$$

The *power density at the receiver* (P_{rec}) is the power density reflected by the target times the loss caused by absorption by the atmosphere.

$$P_{rec} = P_{ref} * T \qquad \text{(Equation 8.6)}$$

The combination of these terms is used to calculate the power that arrives at the receiver in order to predict how much power must be transmitted to obtain a useful measurement. The process of actually calculating the distance measured hinges on the type of measurement technique used. There are two major techniques—pulsed laser measurements and cw laser measurements.

8.2.1 Pulsed Laser Techniques

To measure distance using a pulsed laser involves sending a pulse to the target and measuring the time it takes to return to the receiver. The pulse is often generated using a Q-switch (see Chapter 4). The departure of the pulse is synchronized with a digital electronic counter that begins as the pulse leaves. The counter then stops when the pulse reaches the receiver. As shown in Figure 8-8, it is important that the start and stop of the counter be synchronized at the same position on the pulse.

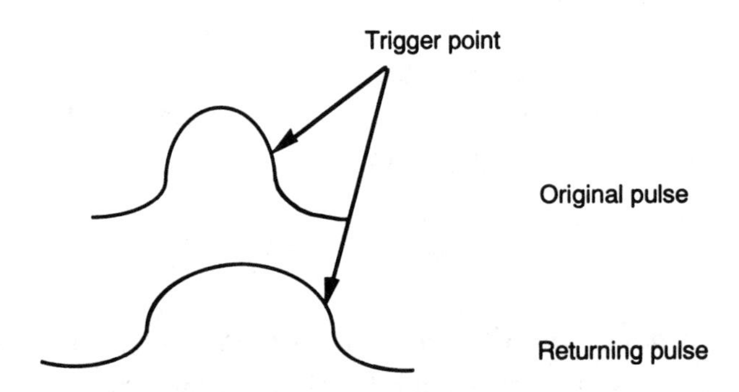

Figure 8-8 Pulses in distance measurement

It is important to notice that the shape of the pulse will be changed by the time it returns to the receiver. This change in shape can lead to errors in the distance measurement unless the detecting circuitry of the receiver is modified to accommodate for it.

8.2.2 Continuous Wave Laser Techniques

The beam from a cw laser can be used to measure distance as well. The beam is modulated by an external oscillator connected to the laser's power supply or placed in the path of the beam (see Chapter 4 for more on modulation). The phase of the original beam is then compared to the phase of the returning beam. In a principle similar to interferometry, the time it took the beam to make the round trip (t_r) is calculated from the phase difference (ϕ) and the frequency of the modulating signal (f) using

$$t_r = \phi/(2\pi f) \qquad \text{(Equation 8.7).}$$

Figure 8-9 shows a common setup for a cw distance measurement system. The modulation is provided by an acousto-optic device, and the original signal is obtained by a beam splitter placed in the path of the outgoing laser beam.

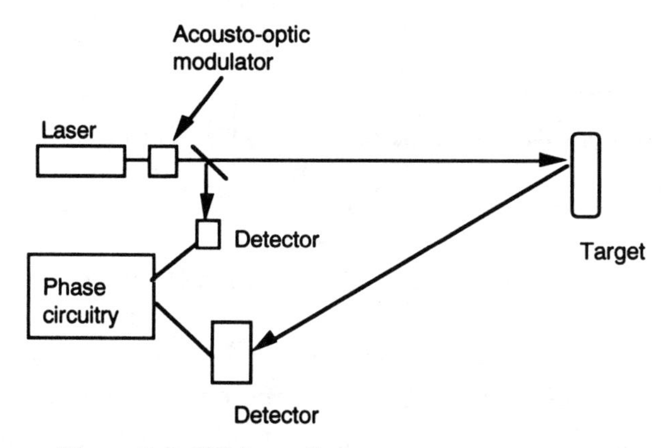

Figure 8-9 CW laser distance measurement system

The returning beam is detected and the phase of the two signals is compared with a circuit that also makes the calculation to determine the round trip time.

8.3 Spectroscopy

Spectroscopy is a method of analysis that uses the physical separation of light. Spectroscopy can be used to analyze a light source, determine the types and concentration of elements and compounds in an unknown chemical through light absorption, or to detect a light signal in the presence of other electromagnetic radiation. Of the three, the use of spectroscopy in analyzing chemicals is where lasers are used most. In fact, the phrase *laser spectroscopy* is generally used to describe this type of analysis.

A device used for spectroscopy is known as a spectrometer, and often the area of the spectrum used by the spectrometer is attached to its name. For example, a spectrometer that uses ultraviolet (UV) and visible (VIS) light for analysis is known as a UV/VIS spectrometer;, while one that uses infrared light (IR) is known as an IR spectrometer.

As shown in Figure 8-10, the basic spectrometer used for chemical analysis consists of a light source, a sample of the chemical, and a detector.

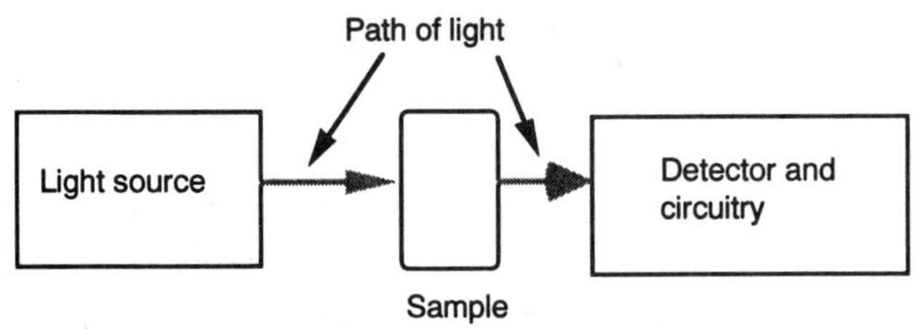

Figure 8-10 Block diagram of a spectrometer

As the light from the source passes through the sample, some of it is absorbed. The detector measures the amount of light that is absorbed and records it. By using several wavelengths of light, a characteristic curve of the absorption vs. wavelength is created for the sample (see Figure 8-11). This curve is then compared to curves made with samples of known composition and concentration to determine what chemicals, and their concentration, are contained in the source.

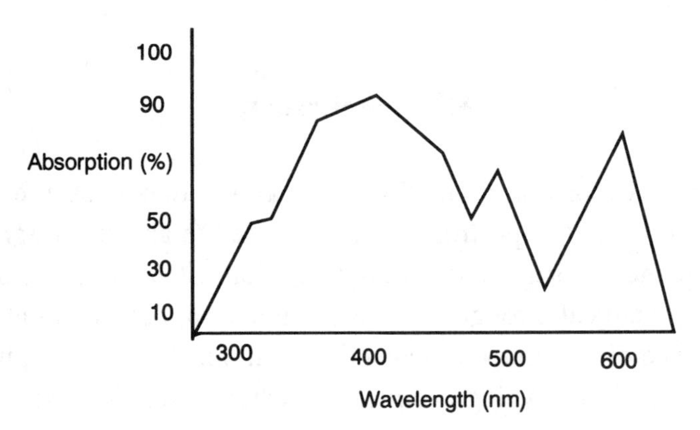

Figure 8-11 Common curve generated by a spectrometer

8.3.1 Principles of Operation

The theory of absorption spectroscopy is based upon two laws—Lambert's Law and Beer's Law. Lambert's law (also known as the exponential law of absorption) states that the amount of light absorbed by a material increases exponentially with the size of the material. Figure 8-12 illustrates the effect of thickness on absorption. Notice that the absorption does not increase linearly (in a straight line) but curves in an exponential fashion.

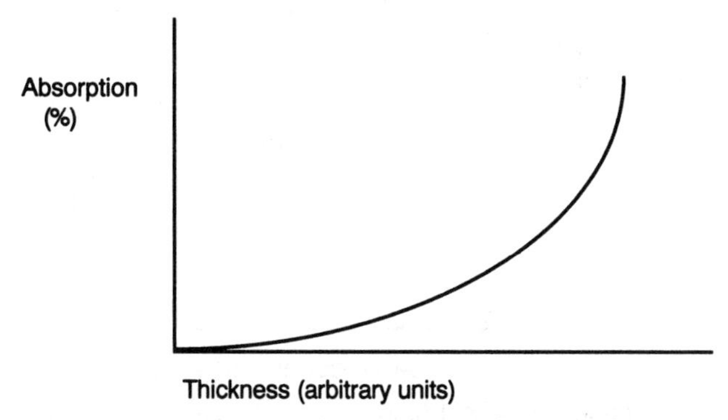

Figure 8-12 Absorption as a function of thickness

Beer's law relates the absorption of a chemical to its concentration. Like thickness, concentration increases the absorption exponentially. The effects of concentration would be similar to the effects for thickness shown in Figure 8-12.

In addition to Beer's law and Lambert's law, spectroscopy is based on the fact that each element or compound absorbs a unique set of wavelengths. The absorption spectrum (the range of wavelengths absorbed) of an element or compound is a direct result of its energy levels (see Chapter 1).

The spectrometer uses the principles of Beer's law, Lambert's law and the absorption spectrum to identify the types of chemicals (qualitative analysis) and their concentration (quantitative analysis) in an unknown sample. To measure the quantity, a calibration curve is created by measuring the absorption of a known chemical at different concentrations. The resulting graph is shown in Figure 8-13 and is sometimes known as a Beer's Law Plot. When the absorption of an unknown sample is measured, the results are compared to the calibration curve to determine the concentration.

To identify the chemicals in a sample (qualitative), the absorption spectra of several known chemicals are prepared by passing several different wavelengths through them and recording which wavelengths are absorbed. These spectra can then be compared to the wavelengths absorbed by an unknown sample to identify the chemicals it contains.

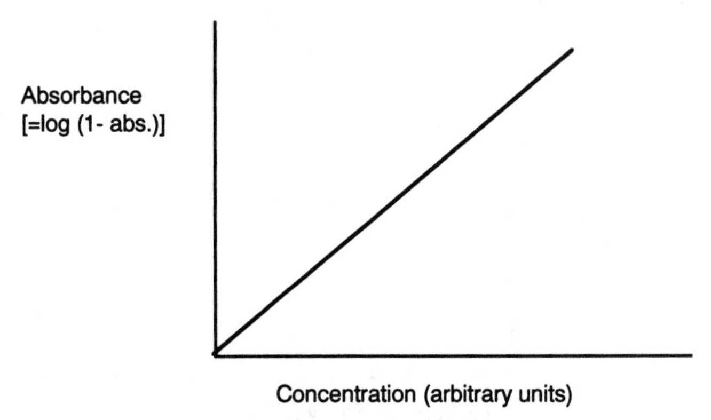

Figure 8-13 Calibration curve or Beer's Law Plot
(the absorbance is the log of the absorption)

8.3.2 Common Design

The spectrometer consists of a light source that allows selection of specific wavelengths, a sample holder, detection circuitry, and a data output device. The light source can be one of several setups including broad-band (several wavelengths) sources equipped with a wavelength selection device such as a prism or grating. However, the light source that is of most interest in this book is a laser. Since the light source is required to provide several wavelengths of light, only a few lasers are applicable. Of these, the most common is a tunable dye laser. Recall from Chapter 2 that the dye laser is made from an organic dye which is pumped by a light source (either a lamp or another laser) and will produce a laser beam at several wavelengths. The exact wavelengths produced by the dye laser will depend on the type of dye used and the type of pumping source. By using a set pumping source and changing dyes, it is possible to obtain wavelengths that range from near ultraviolet through the visible spectrum and even out to near infrared. Figure 8-14 shows a typical laser spectrometer.

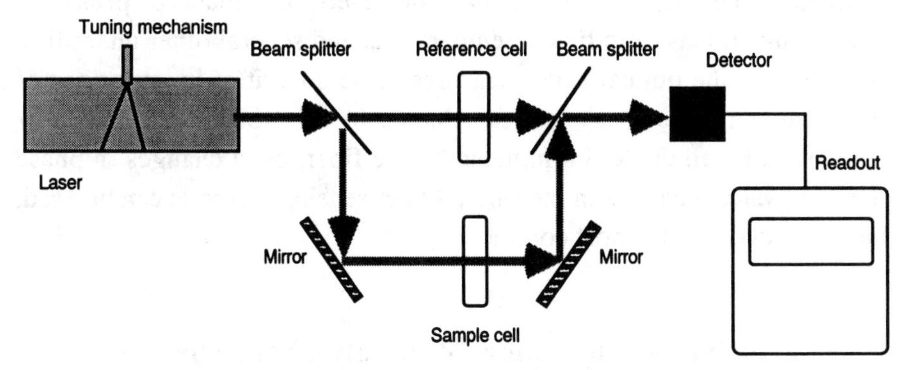

Figure 8-14 Laser spectrometer

The laser beam is split into two parts. One half the beam passes through the sample contained in a quartz cell. The other half of the beam passes through a reference cell that is used to negate the absorption effects of the cell and the solvent that is used to dissolve the sample chemical. Both beams are recombined at the detector which measures the absorption and passes the signal to a readout device.

8.3.3 Applications

The laser spectrometer is used to analyze chemicals that are unknown through absorption effects as discussed above or through the process of fluorescence. Fluorescence is an effect that occurs in some materials when they absorb light. Instead of converting the light to atomic energy, fluorescent material re-emits the light at another wavelength. This new light can be analyzed to determine the properties of the sample material. Because of the laser's monochromatic beam, it can produce a highly accurate analysis, and the beam's high irradiance allows for testing of larger concentrations.

8.4 Fiber-Optic Sensors

The optical fiber is discussed as a communications medium in Chapter 6. In addition to this application, optical fibers are often used as sensors. The optical fiber can be used to measure pressure, displacement, magnetic fields, temperature, and several other quantities. As a sensor, the optical fiber measures these quantities in variations of light intensity due to a physical change in the fiber or reflection or absorption by an object illuminated by the fiber, or in changes in phase due to physical changes in the fiber. Other sensing methods can be used, but these two are the most common.

8.4.1 Principles of Operation—Intensity Change Sensors

The change in intensity of the light in a fiber can be caused by reflection or absorption of an object illuminated by the fiber. This type of sensor involves two fibers, one of which carries the light to the object and one that returns the light to a detector. Figure 8-15 shows a sensor used to measure position through reflection and a sensor used to measure concentration through absorption.

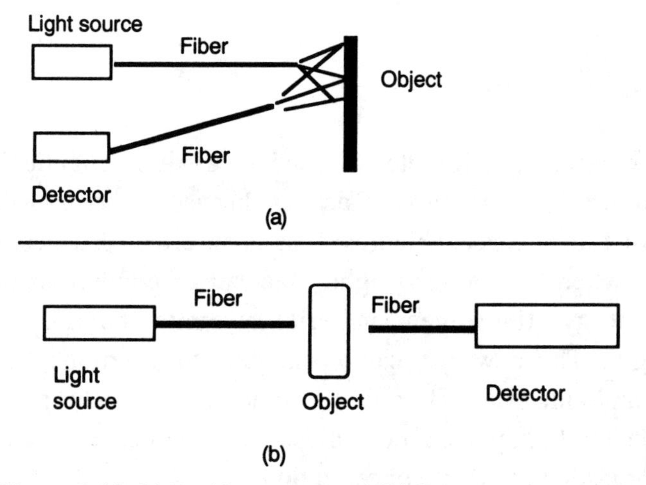

Figure 8-15 **(a)** Position sensor and **(b)** Concentration sensor

The position sensor routes light through a fiber toward the object. The object reflects the light toward another fiber which routes it back to a detector. Changes in the position of the object will result in changes in the amount of reflection received at the detector. The concentration sensor passes light from one fiber through a material to another fiber. The second fiber is connected to a detector which measures the amount of light the material absorbs. Changes in the concentration of the material will cause changes in the absorption.

Changes in light intensity can also be caused by changes in the physical shape of the fiber. In Figure 8-16, a fiber is wedged between two plates. The force of pressure on the top plate will cause bends in the fiber which will lead to loss of light (known as microbend losses).

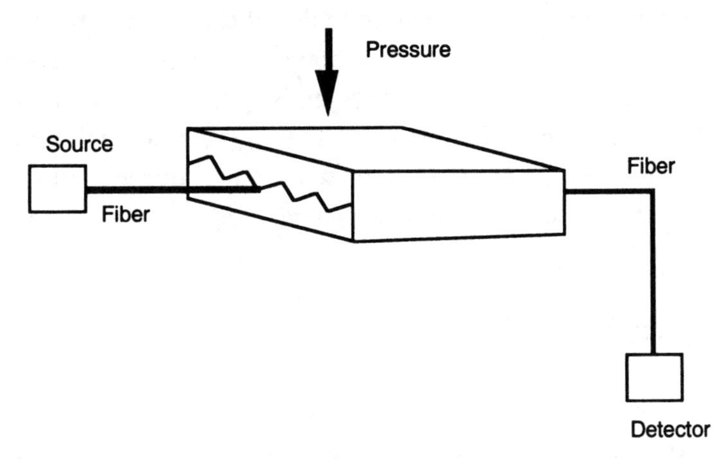

Figure 8-16 Pressure sensor

8.4.2 Principles of Operation—Phase Change Sensors

A change in the length of fiber can cause a change in the phase of the light passing through it (see Chapter 3 and section 8.1). The phase change sensor uses this principle to detect things like temperature and magnetic fields. In Figure 8-17 a phase change sensor for measuring temperature is shown. As the sensor is heated, the fiber grows longer and introduces a phase shift. The combination of the light in the sensor fiber and the light in the reference fiber will cause interference effects at the detector. These interference effects change with the phase change.

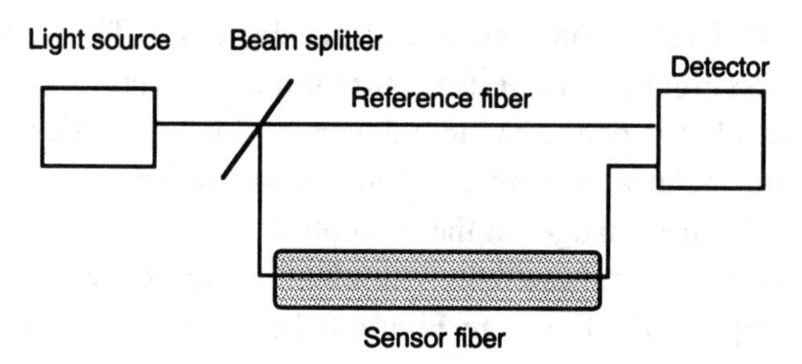

Figure 8-17 Temperature Measurement

Phase change can also be used to detect changes in orientation, as with a fiber-optic gyroscope. A fiber-optic gyroscope (FOG) consists of a single fiber in a large coil. A laser beam is split into two parts sent into both ends of the fiber. If the coil is rotated (even a small amount) a phase change between the two beams will be introduced, and when the beams recombine, there will be interference effects.

8.4.3 Applications

Fiber-optic sensors are used in a wide range of applications. The concentration sensor is used in the exhaust of some cars to monitor emissions and provide feedback to the electronic circuit that controls the engine. Fiber-optic gyroscopes are used in navigation systems in cars and aboard ships.

Fiber-optic systems that measure vibration and pressure are often incorporated into systems known as *smart structures*. The smart structure is made of materials with built-in sensors. The sensors monitor the stress and strain on the structure and provide the information to a central controller, which provides information about the integrity of the structure and may even make adjustments to compensate for excessive stress. Smart structures are used in airplanes to provide warnings about possible failures.

BIBLIOGRAPHY

Bender, Gary. *Principles of Chemical Instrumentation.* Philadelphia: W.B. Saunders Company, 1987.

Hecht, E. and Zajac, A. *Optics.* Reading, Mass.: Addison-Wesley, 1974.

Jenkins, Eugene F. and White, Alfred H. *Fundamentals of Optics.* New York: McGraw-Hill, 1976.

Laser Applications – Volume 8. Waco: Center for Occupational Research and Development, 1990.

Measures, Raymond. "Advances Towards Fiber Optic Based Smart Structures," *Optical Engineering.* volume 31, no. 1, January, 1992.

O'Shea, Donald. *Elements of Modern Optical Design.* New York: John Wiley & Sons, 1985.

Zanger, Henry and Cynthia. *Fiber Optics Communications and Other Applications.* New York: Macmillan Publishing Company, 1991.

Unit III

TROUBLESHOOTING AND MAINTAINING LASERS

The necessary maintenance and troubleshooting of lasers will change (in the skills required, level of difficulty and even feasibility) with the type of laser. Unit III divides laser types into three broad categories based on their output power. Traditionally, high power lasers lend themselves to repair more than smaller lasers. The reasons are several, but they include the cost of the laser, the complexity of its operation and the type of components it incorporates. Large lasers tend to be composed of electronics systems, cooling systems and perhaps gas systems that can be repaired and maintained. They are generally expensive devices and warrant this maintenance. Chapter 9 provides a step by step guide for the troubleshooting and installation of high powered gas and solid lasers.

Medium power lasers, while incorporating many of the same devices as high power lasers, are not always as repairable. Chapter 10 describes the process of troubleshooting these lasers. Many of the procedures are the same as high power lasers so references to Chapter 9 are given at appropriate intervals.

Low power lasers are usually much less costly and are sometimes not fixable. Chapter 11 provides more information on beam diagnosis, power sources and operation for the two main low power lasers -- the helium neon and the semiconductor.

Repair work on lasers increases the ever present dangers involved and no attempts should be made to perform any of the steps discussed in this unit without a solid foundation in laser safety.

Appendix C gives detailed information on this topic. Also, the information given in this unit is based on commonly accepted procedures, but it should never supersede the manufacturer's guidelines for your laser.

9

HIGH-POWER AND INDUSTRIAL LASERS

Introduction

This chapter is a reference guide for the troubleshooting and installation of typical high-power and industrial laser systems. The installation guidelines are in step-by-step form so that the reader can follow the procedure sequentially. Similarly, the troubleshooting information is presented in flowchart form so you may quickly locate a specific symptom, diagnose the possible problem, and discover the cure. A general description of the component or system at fault, and procedures for correcting the problem, are included. However, the manufacturer's suggestions for repair of the specific laser system you are troubleshooting should be followed whenever possible. Troubleshooting of gas discharge lasers (such as the carbon dioxide) and solid-state lasers (such as the Nd:YAG) is covered in section 9.1. Installation procedures for these two laser types are provided in sections 9.2 and 9.3.

9.1 Troubleshooting Gas Discharge and Solid-State Lasers

The following flowchart is provided for helping to locate the symptom of interest and its potential problems:

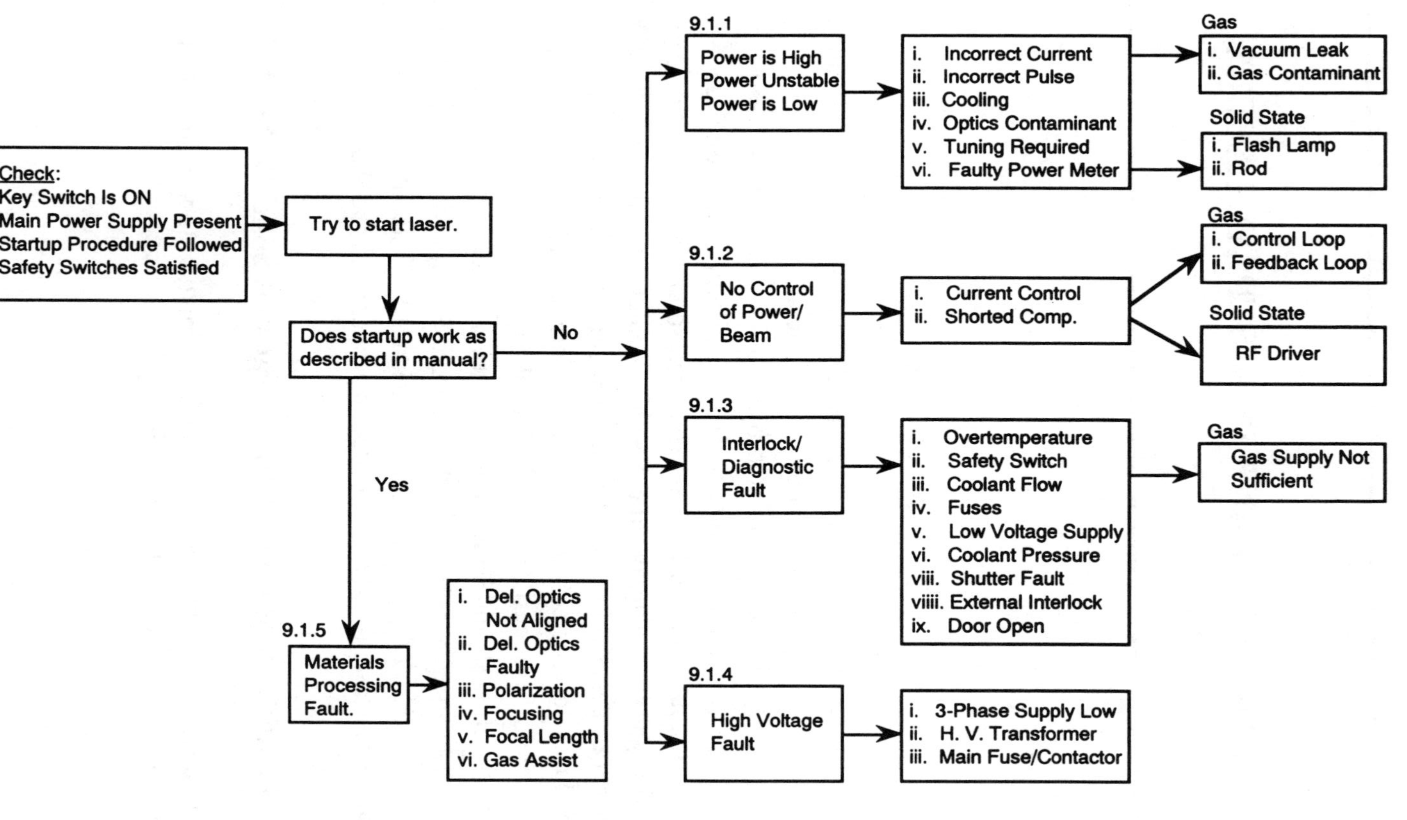

Flow Chart for Troubleshooting High-Power and Industrial Lasers

9.1.1 Power is Low, High, or Unstable

i. Incorrect Current Selected

When power output is too low, too high, or unstable, it is conceivable that an error could have been made by the operator when setting up the desired laser operating parameters. Verifying these parameters is the first step that should be taken to try and pinpoint the reason for the failure condition.

In addition, many of the laser designs currently available include circuitry to allow current level to be selected by a control device external to the laser. If this external device is not sending the correct signals to the laser, the laser output may not be what is expected. Verifying the operation of the controller is accomplished by setting the laser current with the laser's internal controls and noting the output power. If the power is different than when the current is set with the external device, then that device is faulty.

ii. Incorrect Pulse Width

Incorrect pulse width settings can cause power problems. The pulse width settings should be checked, and if the pulse width is controlled by an external device, then the pulse width should be set with the internal laser controls and the resulting power compared to the power from the external controller.

iii. Cooling Circuits Unregulated

All lasers require some form of cooling to extract waste heat from the system. Typically an external chiller is used to provide the laser with a temperature-stable water supply at a fixed pressure and flow. Some lasers require that the water also contain corrosion inhibitors, antifreeze, or other additives. In general, lasers have sensors that monitor the coolant and either warn the operator or shut off the laser if the pressure, temperature, or flow are outside the required parameters. It is possible that these sensors may malfunction, allowing the laser to overheat and causing the output power to drop.

If the sensors indicate a cooling problem or the laser is excessively hot, the pressure, temperature, and flow of the coolant should be checked. The chiller may be supplying an inadequate amount of coolant or coolant at too high a temperature.

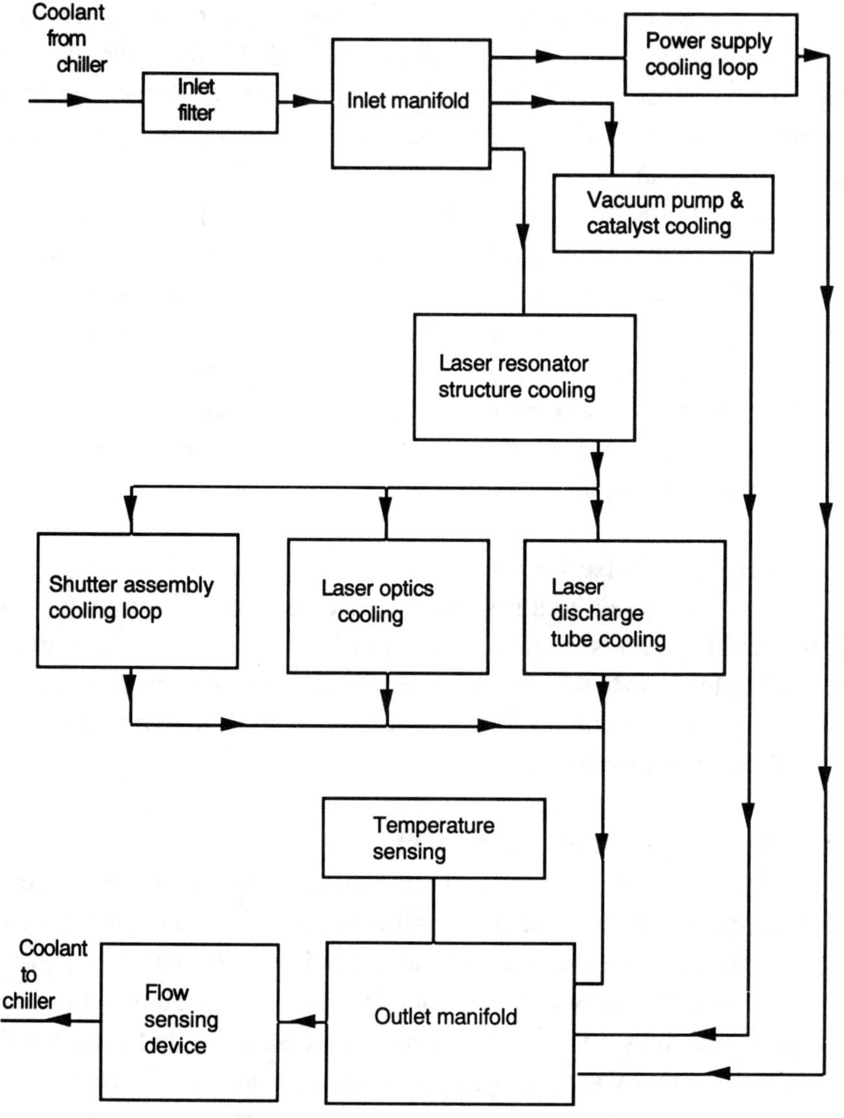

Figure 9-1 Typical coolant circuit

iv. Optics Contaminated

In normal laser operation, optics contamination should not be a problem. However, if the circulating gas is not being filtered properly, contamination can result from blowers or pumps used in circulating the gas. If optics contamination is discovered, the filters for these devices should be checked and replaced if necessary.

Contaminated optics can be identified by close inspection. Observing light—from a pen light or similar source—as it is transmitted through the mirror or lens can reveal foreign particles on the surface. Light that shines at a glancing angle to the surface of the mirror or lens can also reveal contamination.

Cleaning optics is a delicate procedure since their surfaces can be damaged easily. Great care should be taken throughout the operation. The manufacturer will provide guidelines for cleaning the optics and these should be followed meticulously. In general, the surface is cleaned with a reagent like methanol or acetone. Lens cleaning tissue is used to apply the cleaner. The surface of the lens or mirror should never be wiped with a dry tissue, and tissues should be disposed of after one pass over the surface. Often, canned "clean air" is used to remove dust and other particles before the cleaner is applied.

v. Laser Requires Tuning

Tuning or aligning the laser involves adjusting the position and angle of the output coupler and high reflectance mirrors. Regular tuning is not necessary, but if the mirrors have been replaced or moved they may need to be realigned.

Mirrors are typically mounted in a block with differentially threaded tuning screws that adjust the tilt of the mirrors. Some lasers also have motor driven adjustments so the mirrors can be aligned without opening the protective housing. The manufacturer will provide guidelines for mirror alignments. Typically, the mirrors can be aligned by initially using an autocollimator or a low-powered laser beam that is mounted in line with the mirrors. The alignment can be fine tuned by tweaking the tuning screws while observing the output power. Mirrors would be adjusted for the maximum power output. Great care should be taken if the laser is operated with protective housing removed, since extreme high voltage and laser radiation hazards exist in the cavity. Lasers are equipped with interlocks so they will not normally operate with the housing removed. Defeating these interlocks is extremely dangerous and should only be attempted by an experienced laser technician taking the appropriate safety precautions, which includes wearing protective goggles.

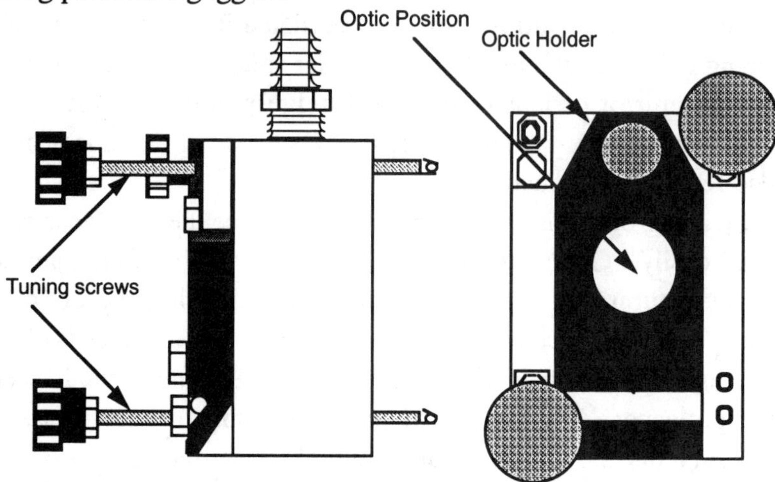

Figure 9-2 Typical mirror mount

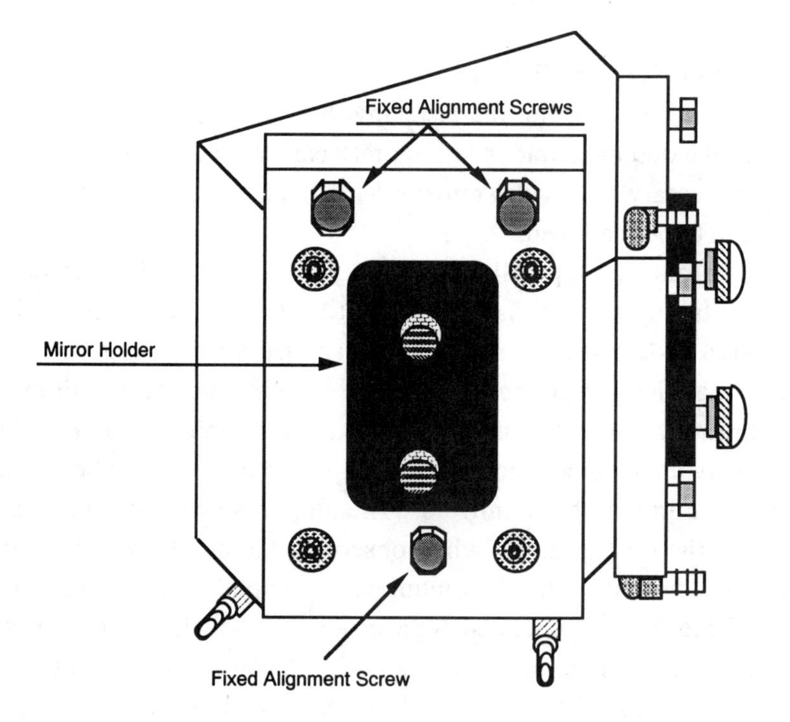

Figure 9-3 Typical beam folding block

vi. Power Meter Faulty

If all other options have been eliminated, it is possible that the power meter is faulty and giving incorrect readings. The power of the laser can be checked with an external measuring device such as a calorimeter.

GAS DISCHARGE LASERS

i. Vacuum Leak is Present

Industrial carbon dioxide lasers typically circulate the lasing gas in a partial pressure. The lasing gas is a mixture of nitrogen, helium, and carbon dioxide. The ratio of these three gasses is important. If a vacuum leak is present, air will be introduced into the laser, contaminating the circulating gas with excess nitrogen. The result will be a decrease in power and possible pulse skipping in pulse operation.

If a vacuum leak is present, the pressure of the laser will be affected. It may take the system longer to reach the proper pressure or the pressure may be higher than normal. The pressure of the system should be checked to see if it is at the recommended level. Leaks in the system will make it more difficult for the vacuum pump to reach the required pressure, and mechanical pumps will sound different when they labor harder to produce a vacuum. To determine the location if a leak is present, all connections in the system should be checked for visible cracks, holes, or other sources of leaks. Smaller leaks can be located by making a solution of soap and water and dabbling it on the vacuum lines and fittings. Small bubbles in the solution indicate holes that cause leaks. Leaks in connectors or lines can be fixed by replacing the faulty part.

ii. Gas Contaminated

Laser manufacturers specify a required gas purity (a typical requirement might be 99.995% pure with a hydrocarbon and moisture content of less than ten parts per million). These requirements must be strictly adhered to or power may be reduced and optics' lifetime may be degraded. Most gas vendors have "laser purity" gasses or similar products for meeting the specified requirements.

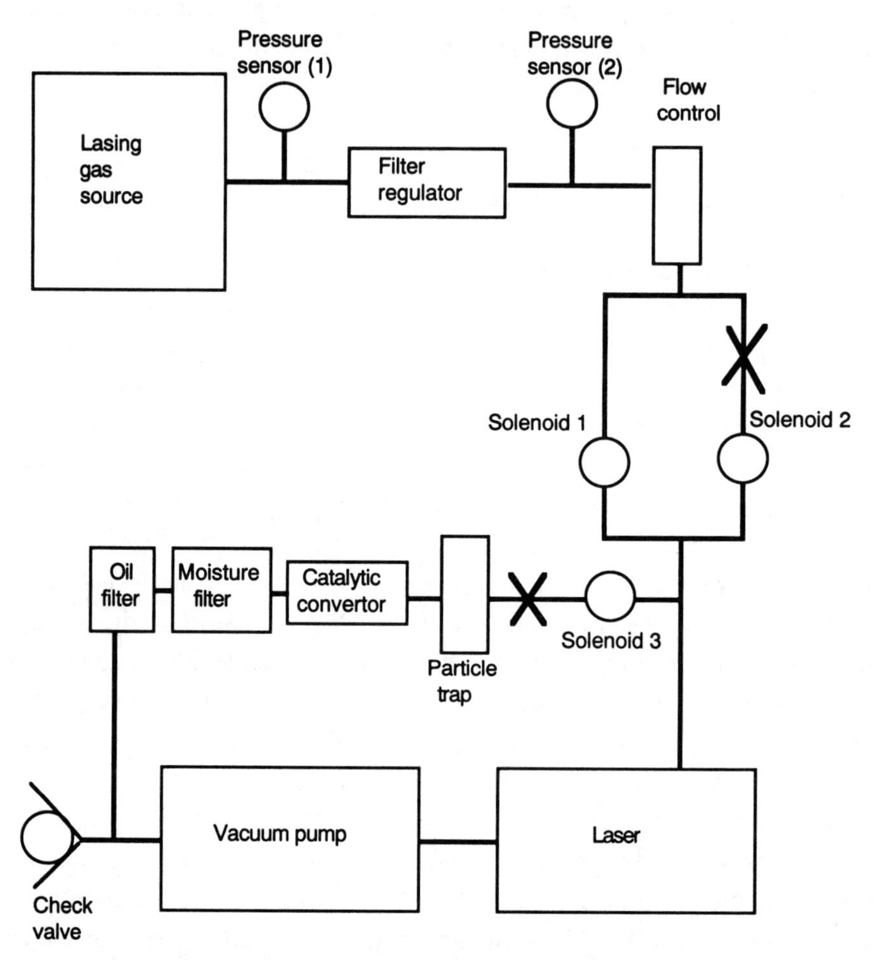

Pressure sensors 1 and 2 are used to sense when the gas supply is becoming low or has been exhausted. The filter regulator sets a stable input pressure to the flow control valve, which is set to determine a known flow into the laser. The three valves, solenoids 1, 2, and 3 are used to determine if the laser is to be run on fresh or recycled gas and are controlled typically by a microprocessor unit. The oil filter, moisture filter, catalyst and particle filter, are the main components in the Gas Recycler Unit. The vacuum pump draws gas around the laser and exhausts to the check valve, which supplies a back pressure to force gas through the recycler.

Figure 9-4 Typical gas circuit—slow flow laser

SOLID STATE

i. Lamp Degraded or Not Functioning

Over a period of time the lamp in a solid-state laser will degrade. As its output power decreases, the strength of the beam decreases as well. Lamps may also experience catastrophic failure (they explode) as a result of the current increasing too rapidly or of improper installation. Lamps should be replaced when their degradation reaches the point where the desired beam power is no longer obtainable. Manufacturers generally recommend replacement after a specified number of hours of operation or after a specified number of shots.

Replacing the lamp requires removal of the old lamp by loosening any mounting brackets or clips and any seals for containing coolant. If the lamp has exploded, any shards of glass should be carefully removed with a cotton swab or a rolled up piece of lens tissue. The replacement lamp must be mounted properly so that its electrical connections are correct. If the anode and cathode of the lamp are reversed, the lamp may explode when the laser is restarted. Anode and cathode are generally identified by the lamp manufacturer and the laser manufacturer. The anode of the lamp is usually rounded in shape, while the cathode is pointed. Lamps should be carefully cleaned before installation.

ii. Rod Damaged

Although the laser rod is not normally subject to degradation like the lamp, it may suffer damage through rough handling or if the coolant is contaminated. A damaged rod will have visible flaws such as cracks or chips or may have a coating due to contaminated coolant.

Replacing the rod is similar to replacing the lamp, except that the rod has no electrical connections and is usually not installed with a specific orientation. Great care should be taken when handling the rod since it is an optical component. Oils from the skin can contaminate the surface of the rod and reduce its performance.

9.1.2 No Control of Power/Beam

i. No Current Control in Discharge

Failure of the control loop or feedback loop may lead to lack of current control in the laser discharge. In either case, failures may be associated with high voltage transformers, saturable reactors, or some other control type device, such as power transistors or triode valves. It is beyond the scope of this guide to offer advice on fault finding of high voltage circuits, if only because of the safety concerns involved, and if a problem of this nature would arise, the laser manufacturer should always be contacted first.

ii. Shorted Components

One way to check problems in areas of the power supply where hazardous voltages may normally be present is to check with the input power source disconnected from the laser. Under these conditions, and having followed the manufacturer's normal recommendations for safe operating practice, it will be possible to remove and inspect, visually and electrically, many of the power supply components. Components such as transistors may be checked for shorted junctions, and other passive components in the high voltage circuits such as resistors may be readily confirmed to be of the correct value, using the appropriate measuring equipment. Be prepared on many designs to measure high resistances. Sensing of high voltage values is typically handled by high value resistors in the 100-megaohms or greater range.

General Hints for Component Checking and Verification

Resistors

If the value of a resistor needs to be checked, it should be first ascertained what the expected value is in the circuit. This can be done by referring to the laser manufacturer's schematic and looking for the resistor value as marked. Alternatively, the value can be obtained by reading the resistor's color coding if available. Some resistors may have the value marked on them directly in digits, rather than in color code.

When an expected value has been determined, measure the resistor using a standard digital voltmeter. If the resistor is supposed to have a value higher than 20 MΩ, then a special meter may be required.

If, upon measurement, the value is not as expected, then lift one end of the resistor out of the circuit and check again. This should be done to ensure that measurement is being made only on a single resistor and not two or more resistors in parallel.

Diodes

A diode passes current in only one direction. To test a diode, a reading may likewise be obtained in one direction only. Typical values on a standard meter, for standard diodes, using the "diode check" range, are a reading of 0.7 Ω forward direction and infinite or open in reverse. As with resistors, if the diode checks bad, one end should be lifted from the circuit and the diode re-checked before being replaced.

Capacitors

Some voltmeters include a range for checking capacitance values, but in most cases it may be necessary to use a specially designed meter to check the component value. As with resistors and diodes, removing a component from the circuit may be necessary.

Transistors

These devices may be checked using the diode check range of the meter and conducting a forward and reverse check across the base-emitter, base-collector, and emitter-collector junctions. Some advanced meters and oscilloscopes may include transistor check facilities that are built in.

Integrated Circuits and Microprocessors

Testing of these devices is usually limited to verifying that the correct input voltage/signal is being supplied to the device and then checking that the correct output voltage/signal is being received back from it. Beyond this, refer to the laser supplier or replace the relevant device with a new one.

GAS DISCHARGE

i. Control Loop Faulty

Typical lasers have a control loop that is a circuit for control of current. The gas discharge used in a laser has negative impedance characteristics and will try to draw unlimited current. The control loop allows the power supply to regulate available current and avoid excess current draining by the gas discharge. The control function can be achieved in various ways, but all designs involve a detection circuit or device that will inhibit or shut down the laser operation in the case of excessive current.

ii. Feedback Loop Faulty

A major element of the control loop will be a feedback circuit that is typically used to monitor the status of current and/or voltage on the laser discharge tubes themselves. It is important when operating the laser that all discharge lanes actually ionize when commanded. If they do not all ionize, or if only some ionize, then this condition needs to be detected and reported to the operator as a fault. If all tubes do not ionize, then there will be no laser power output, a condition that is normally sensed and reported routinely. If only some tubes ionize, then power output will be low and it may be impossible to carry out the desired laser application. On DC excited lasers, this situation, if allowed to continue unchecked, can result in laser discharge tubes running at different levels of high voltage and place a great stress on components in the high voltage section of the power supply.

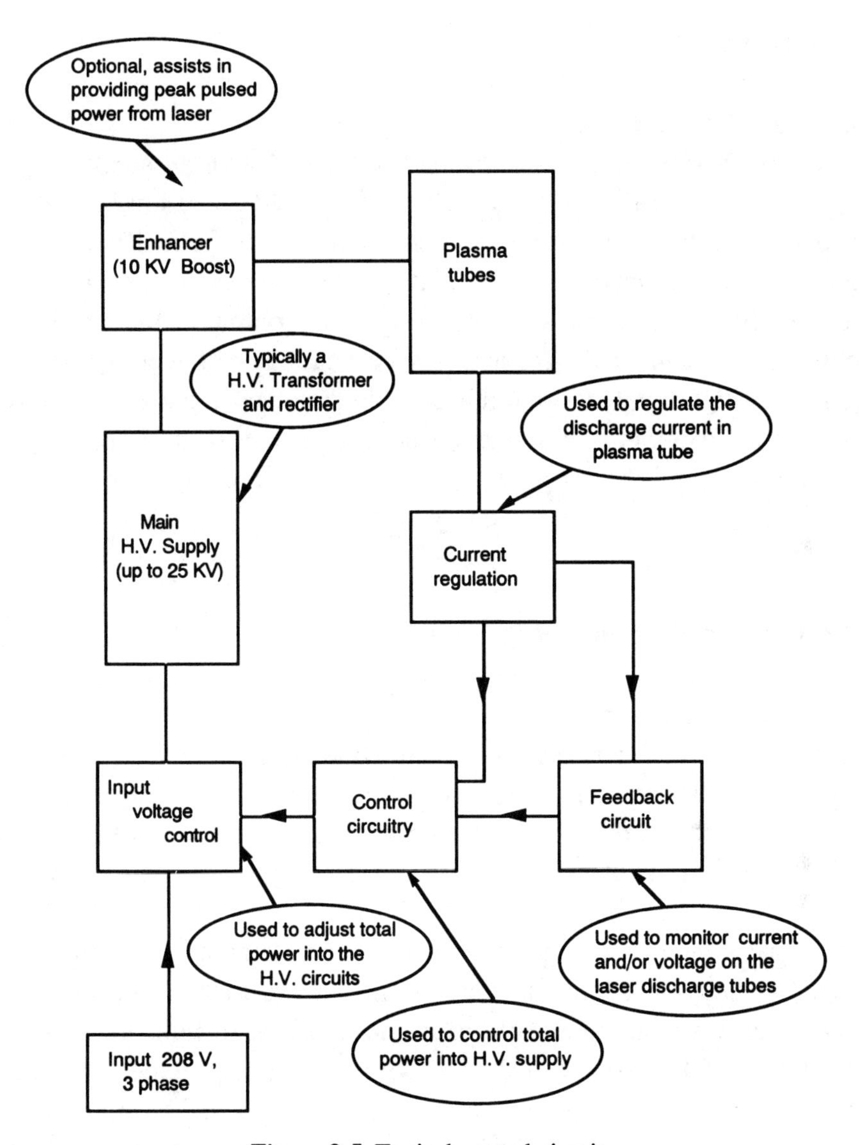

Figure 9-5 Typical control circuit

SOLID STATE

i. RF Driver Fault

For a solid-state laser that is Q-switched with an acousto-optic device, failure in the RF driver will make pulsed operation impossible and may prohibit operating the laser completely. The RF driver is generally a self-contained unit mounted in the laser enclosure. To check the driver, use an oscilloscope to measure the output of the driver and compare it to the manufacturer's specifications. Driver signals are generally high frequency and relatively high voltage signals. No output or a distorted output from the driver indicates it is at fault. Repairing the driver is beyond the scope of this chapter, but simple things such as incoming power, fuses, etc. can be checked.

9.1.3 Interlocks and Diagnostic

i. Overtemperature Conditions

An array of interlocks will be provided to sense whether the laser has reached an overtemperature condition. These may be located at strategic points in the laser and used to sense temperature of air in the cabinet or simply detect water in the cooling loop. Some will be adjustable, others may be fixed. It is not unusual to find several interlocks connected in series, at different points along the path that is being taken by the cooling medium, so that any restriction in flow at any given point will automatically cause an interlock to indicate a failure condition. The laser is a device with a high requirement for heat dissipation, and cooling the laser sufficiently is most important to ensuring long-term operation. For this reason there will probably be more temperature sensors on any laser design than any other type. Sensors may typically be of the type where a contact opens in the event of an overheat and closes again automatically after cooling down. This type of sensor can be checked simply by doing a continuity check using a digital voltmeter.

ii. Safety Switches Active

With power supplies producing voltage levels up to amounts in the thousands of volts and at large currents, safety interlocks are paramount in any laser design. They are typically used on access doors to the laser power supply and on screens in the power supply around high voltage areas. They will also be used on access doors around the area where the laser discharge is being generated. In general, all access doors must be closed to completely satisfy safety interlocks.

iii. Coolant Flow Inadequate

Coolant flow interlocks are incorporated to aid in verifying that the correct flow is being received from the external source provided to the laser. Some systems incorporate water filtration devices at the input to the laser. These filters may become blocked with time, and so reduce flow into the laser machine. The flow sensors will detect this situation and warn the user. See Figure 9-6 for a typical example.

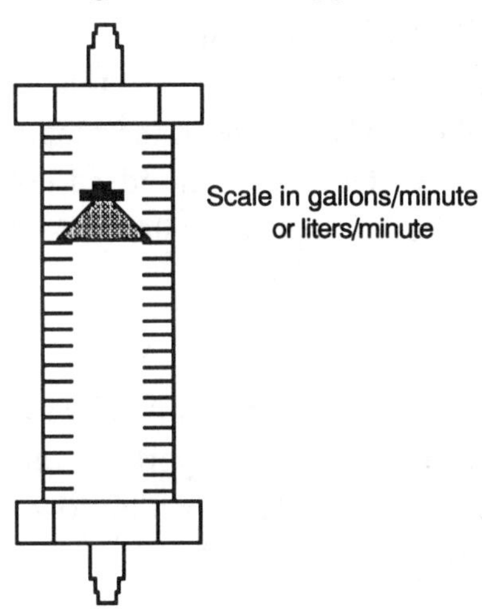

Figure 9-6 Typical flow meter

iv. Fuses Blown

In many cases, circuit breakers have replaced fuses in recent designs. There are times, however, when a fuse is required. The latest power supplies equipped with fuses may well be using the indicator style. These types of fuses incorporate a smaller fuse (in parallel with the main fuse) that has a small spring-loaded plunger device incorporated into it. This device becomes active when the main fuse blows and triggers a microswitch, closing a switch contact and reporting the blown fuse to the laser diagnostic circuits.

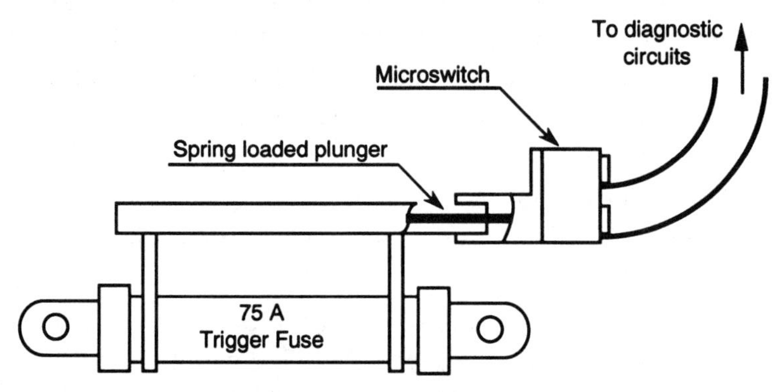

Figure 9-7 Indicator fuse

v. Low Voltage Power Supply Fault

Many interlock and diagnostic circuits are powered by low voltages such as 24 V dc. The failure of the supply will normally result in not being able to start the laser, and indeed not being able to see a diagnostic lamp lit, since the supply for the lamp may be common with the interlock circuit.

vi. Coolant Pressure Inadequate

Inadequate coolant pressure will normally be sensed by a pressure sensitive device installed at the inlet port for the laser cooling water circuit. Operation is similar to that for the flow meter, and detection ranges can normally be set for the device.

vii. Shutter Fault

Modern shutter devices will typically use one or more sensing devices which will perform functions such as overheat sensing, blade position sensing, or coolant flow sensing. Typical shutter designs are either electrically or pneumatically operated devices. Figure 9-8 shows a typical electrically-operated shutter, and Figure 9-9 shows a pneumatically operated design.

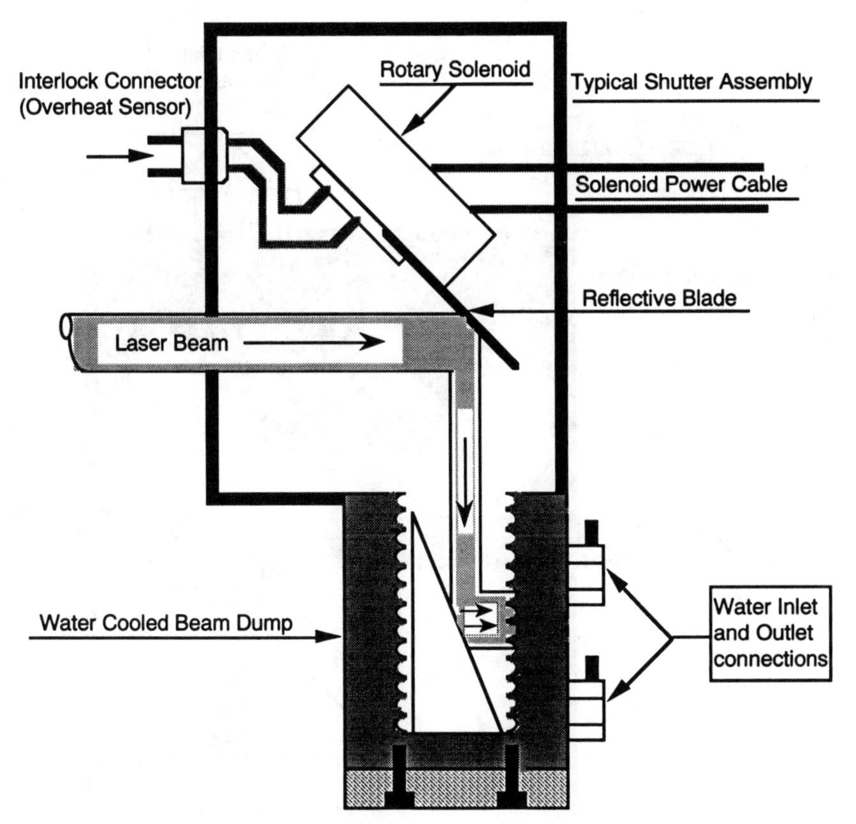

Figure 9-8 Electrically operated shutter

viii. External (Customer) Interlock

This interlock is provided to allow the user some means of shutting the laser down in case of emergency. The interlock is normally wired into the power supply for the main power contactor in the laser. The interlock may be configured such that it can be overridden in the event of service becoming necessary, or may be disabled for safety reasons. A voltage-free contact can be provided to allow the user to simply use a switch to complete the circuit and have control over the laser main power. A typical layout is shown in Figure 9-10.

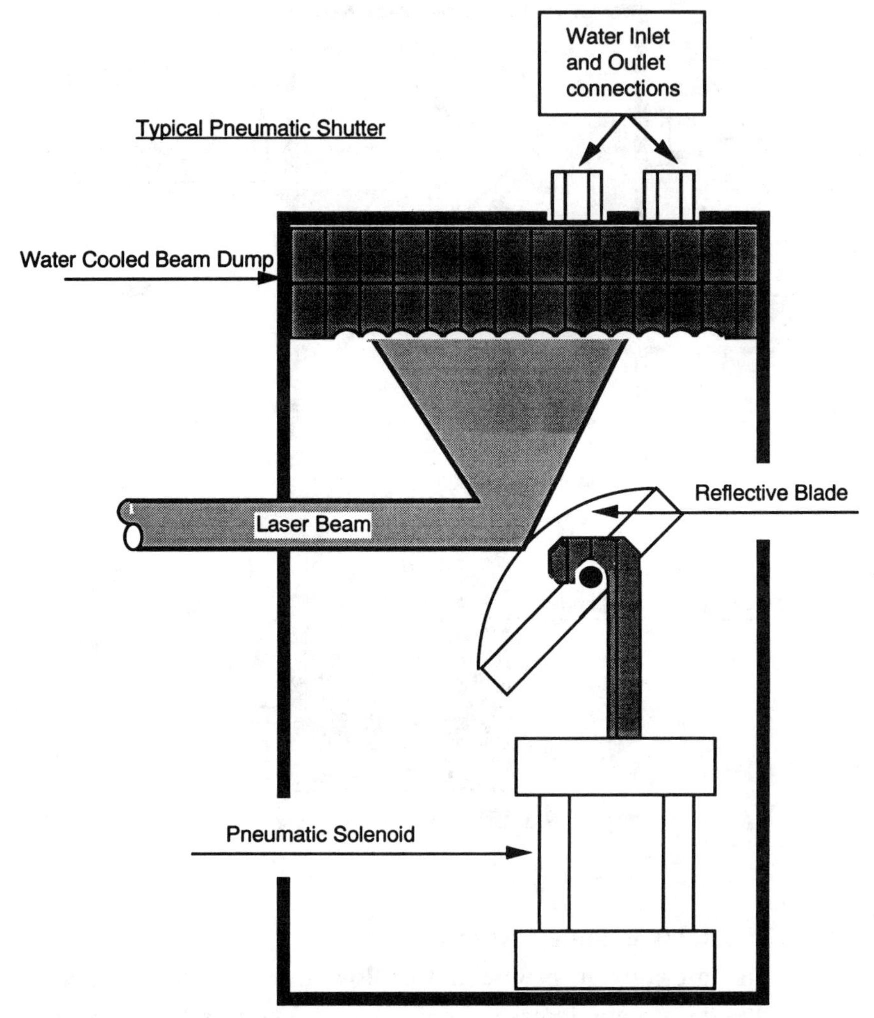

Figure 9-9 Pneumatically operated shutter

ix. Enclosure Door Interlock

The enclosure door interlocks on lasers are provided to prevent accidental exposure to the laser beam, or to the lethal voltages which may be present in the power supply. Opening one of these interlocks will typically disable the power supply or shut the laser main power contactor down.

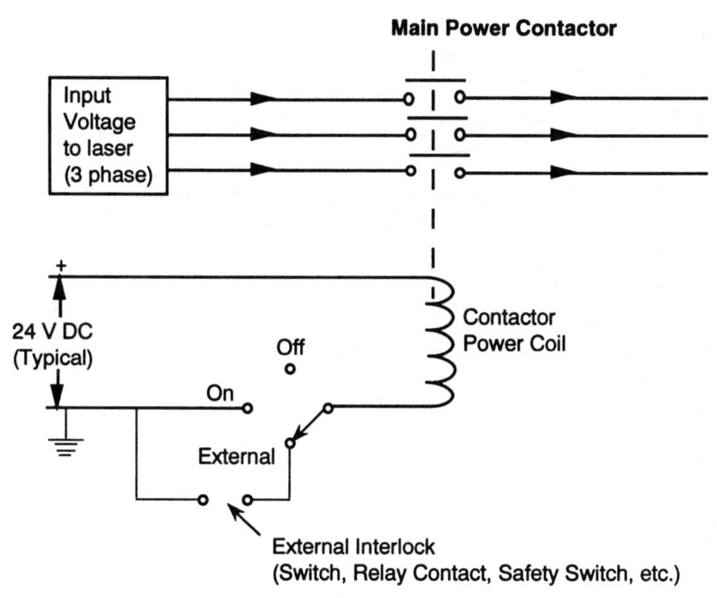

Figure 9-10 Typical external interlock layout

GAS DISCHARGE

i. Gas Supply Not Sufficient

A laser, unless of sealed design, will use a premixed laser gas during normal operation. Recent lasers incorporate two or more interlocks to warn the user of the fact that the laser is about to run out of gas, and that a break in production is imminent. A typical interlock setup may include a first warning when supply pressure drops below a certain value and then a laser shut down at a second set value. The advantage of this system is that the operator has several minutes warning before the second interlock will shut down the laser. Checking of the interlock is normally done by verifying that the input gas pressure specifications provided by the manufacturer have been met. If they have, and the interlock still indicates a fault, then the interlock switch itself needs to be checked (see Figure 9-11).

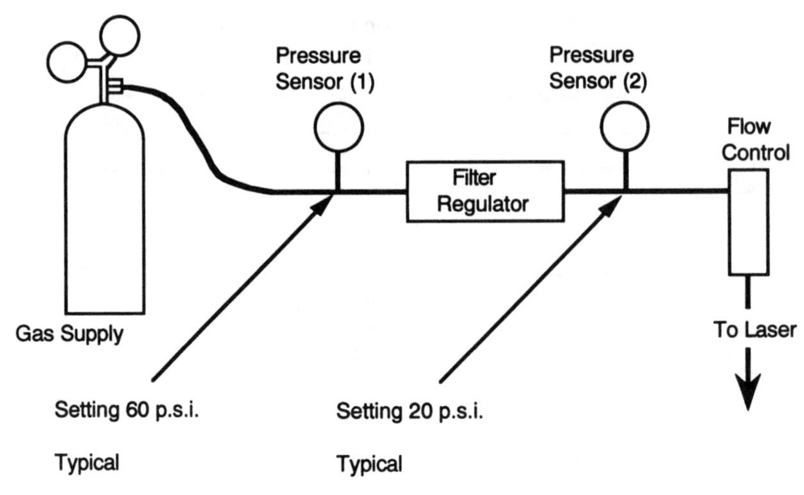

Figure 9-11 Gas supply

9.1.4 Excitation Source Fault

Note: The "Excitation Source" used in a laser may vary with type of machine. Typically, it may be high voltage DC (low current), low voltage DC (high current), or RF (radio frequency). These are the most commonly used. It is beyond the scope of this book to attempt to generalize and offer help in troubleshooting on any of these types of supply, due to the highly hazardous voltages which may be present. If a failure occurs and the supply is suspected to be faulty, the manufacturer should always be contacted prior to attempting repair. The following limited items may assist in localizing the problem.

i. Input Voltage Supply Problem

Most high-power industrial lasers will use a "3-phase" main voltage supply and transform it into a usable excitation source for the lasing medium. In many cases it will be a relatively simple matter to check and verify that a full three of the incoming phases are present at the power input point on the laser. This incoming power can be checked at the main breaker supply to the laser and may be measured using a standard voltmeter. Figure 9-12 shows how to make this check correctly.

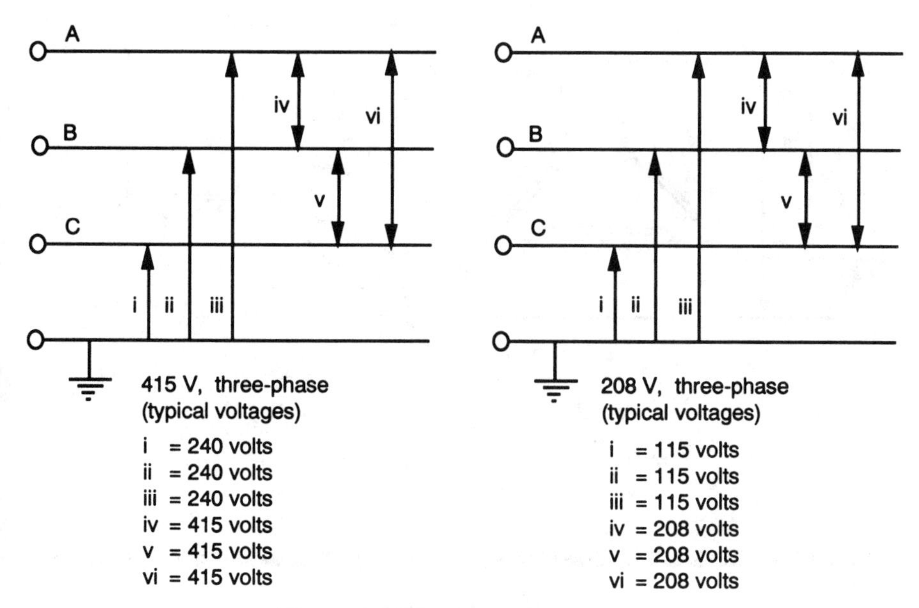

Figure 9-12 Input supply voltages

ii. High Voltage Transformer Failure

Many designs use high voltage as an excitation medium, and failure of a high voltage transformer will prevent operation of the laser. A shorted high voltage transformer will normally result in blown fuses as a primary symptom of failure, and this failure mode is quickly evident to the operator. An open circuit transformer may just demonstrate lower output on its secondary windings, and some supply may be possible from the device, allowing limited operation of the laser. The only checks that can be made safely by an untrained operator are those that can be done with the main power off (see Figure 9-13).

In the example given below, the resistance or inductance of the coils A, B or C can be measured with the system power off. In all cases the readings should be the same for each coil, that is, A = B = C. Typical primary resistances are quite low (10's of ohms) and secondaries are higher (100's of ohms), for step-up high voltage transformers.

It should be stressed that this is only general information and will vary with different laser designs.

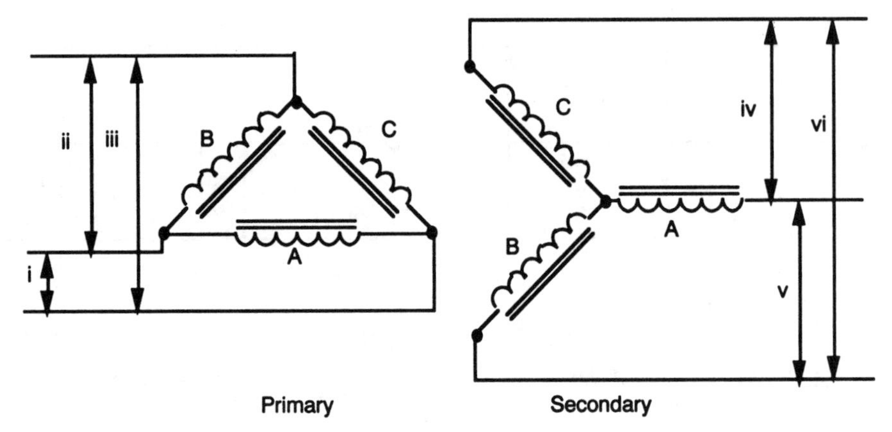

Figure 9-13 Typical three-phase transformer

WARNING

At all times when working around high voltage components, the appropriate safety procedures should be followed. Failure to do so may result in serious injury or death. If in doubt of the correct procedure, contact the equipment manufacturer immmediately.

iii. Fuse or Main Contactor Failure

Each of the above mentioned failures should be pretty simple to verify on most laser systems. For example, the most recent designs of ***Coherent General*** lasers are equipped with diagnostic and interlock circuitry which will report problems to a programmable logic controller, and this in turn can alert the operator to the exact area where the failure has occurred.

9.1.5 Materials Processing Fault

Note: Very often, an initial fault condition with the laser is noticed by the operator because of poor processing results in whatever material is being worked on by the laser. A knowledgeable operator will first seek to verify that the laser is working to the specification and is delivering the requested laser power for the job at hand. If these checks reveal that the laser appears to be functioning correctly, then the operator is left to determine what outside influences may be causing the poor processing results being experienced. The following categories will hold true as potential failure items for most CO_2 laser material processing systems.

i. Beam Delivery Not Aligned

All "beam delivery" systems have the same task to perform, which is to bring the laser beam to bear upon a workpiece. All beam deliveries will usually consist of a set of optical elements which will be used to facilitate the guidance of the laser beam from the laser to a final focusing lens and then to focus the beam onto the material to be processed. The alignment of these optical elements is therefore critical in ensuring that the maximum laser energy is transmitted down the beam delivery to the final focusing lens. A simple beam delivery, using only two optical elements, is shown in Figure 9-12.

Methods for aligning the laser beam so that it is centered down the light tubes, and also centered on the optical elements, are different depending on the system manufacturer. Care must be taken to avoid exposure to the laser beam during the alignment process so, for safety reasons, the manufacturer's guidelines should be followed at all times!

ii. Beam Delivery Optics Faulty

If the optics used in the beam delivery system have become contaminated in any way, they will begin to absorb the incident laser beam, and reduce the total available power that can be delivered to the workpiece. For the operator of the laser, this fault condition will be noticeable in the deterioration of cut quality in the workpiece, even though the laser power meter unit may still be indicating that the required power is actually being supplied from the laser. The precise point at which power is being absorbed by a beam delivery optic can be determined by making a measurement of the laser beam power before and after each optic in the beam delivery. This procedure requires the use of a calorimeter, to measure the power, and is typically carried out by a service technician. Sophisticated power meters, like the ***Coherent Labmaster*** range, can be purchased with sensing devices to assist in aligning the beam and measuring true beam quality.

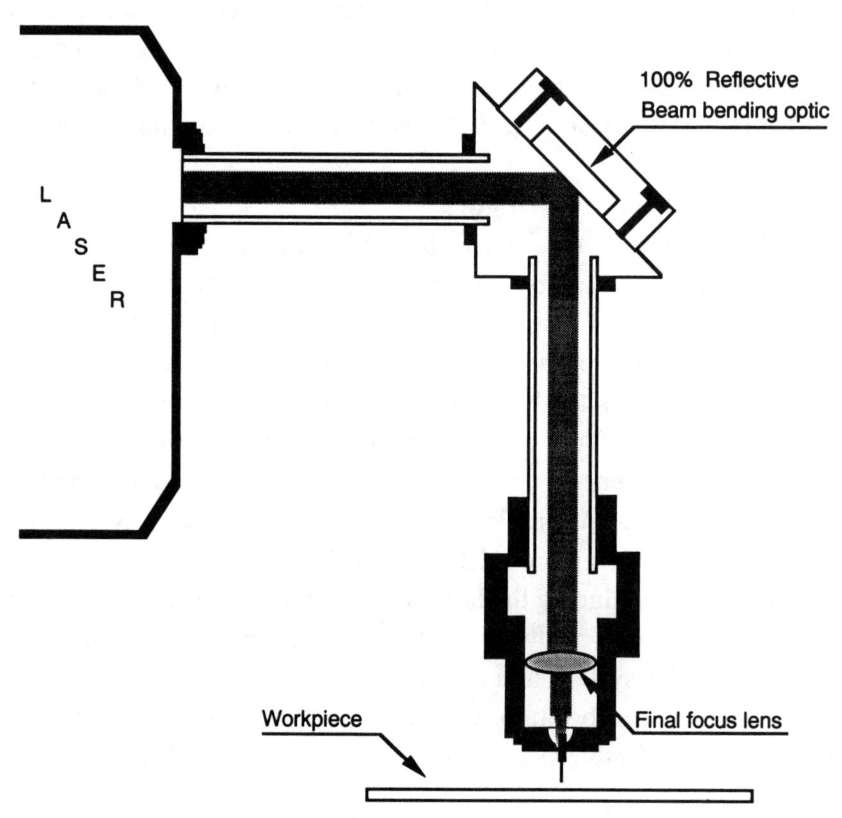

Figure 9-14 Simple beam delivery system

iii. Polarization Fault

Many beam deliveries in use on industrial lasers will incorporate a circular polarizing optic. This device, patented by ***Coherent***, is used to change the laser beam polarization from linearly to circularly polarized. It has been found on certain materials and material thicknesses that a linearly polarized beam will yield unsatisfactory results. This is most easily visible in a piece of thick material that has been cut with a non-circularly polarized beam. The resulting edge quality is as shown in Figure 9-15.

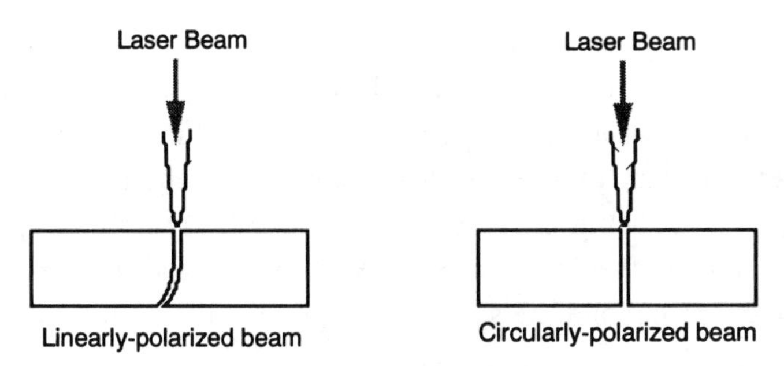

Figure 9-15 Polarization fault
(For purposes of clarity the tapering effect in the above figure has been exaggerated)

Figure 9-16 shows a simple beam delivery with a circular polarizing optic installed. It is recommended that after the polarizing optic, zero phase shift optics only are used. This will ensure the quality of the laser beam at the workpiece.

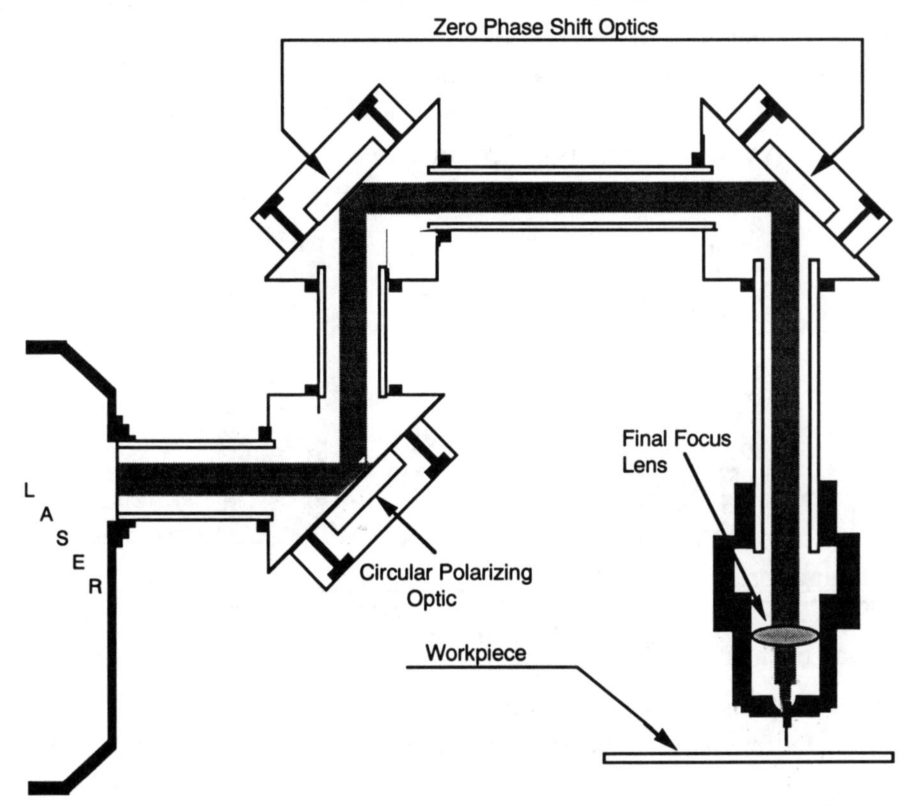

Figure 9-16 Polarizing beam delivery system

iv. Beam Focusing Fault

Correct focusing of the laser beam to the material that is to be processed is critical in achieving a good result. It is recommended that laser users contact their laser manufacturer for help and advice in achieving a good setup of the laser focus point. The reason for this is that the setup of the focus may vary with material and laser power output, and it is beyond the scope of this guide to attempt to list all the possible variables.

v. Lens Focal Length Incorrect for the Material

There is one general rule which can be stated to assist the user in choosing the correct lens for the job at hand, and that is that the thicker the material to be processed, the longer the lens focal length should be. The reason for this is that a beam focused by a 5 inch lens will have a greater depth of field than that of a 1.5 inch lens, and hence will yield a narrower cut width in the material and maintain a higher power density over the depth of the cut. This in turn will ensure a high cut edge quality. An example of this effect can be seen in Figure 9-17.

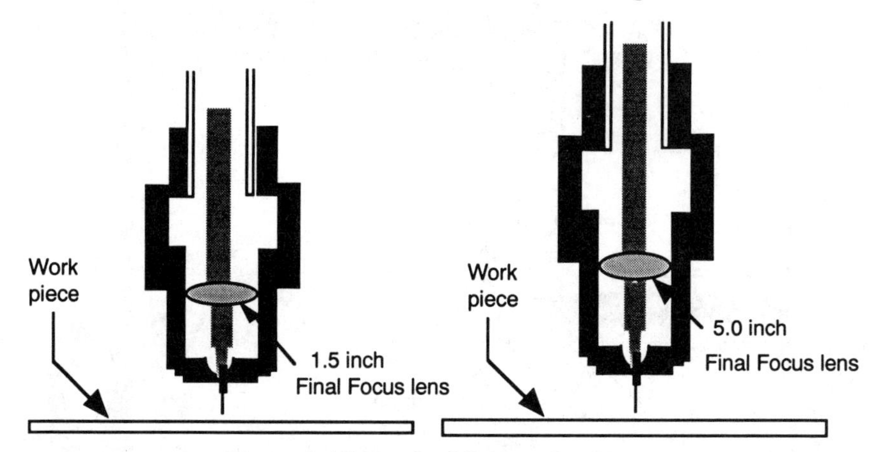

Figure 9-17 Depth of field vs. focal length

vi. Cutting Assist Gas Fault

Different assist gases are used in laser processing with different materials. The type of gas, the pressure at which it should be supplied, and the material most suited, are all variables which should be carefully considered to ensure that the best laser process results are obtained.

Again it is beyond the scope of this guide to attempt to list these variables, and it is suggested that the manufacturer of the laser be contacted for assistance. In fact, many laser builders will be happy to validate for a user whether a laser is suited to the material, and will run the first trials in their own applications laboratory.

9.2 Installing a Solid-State Laser

Information in this section and the next is given in a step-by-step form so that the reader may follow the procedure sequentially. Manufacturer's guidelines should be used for details on the process.

9.2.1 Inspection

•1. Unpack and inspect laser—report any damage to authorized personnel.
•2. Verify parts inventory with parts received.
•3. Read manufacturer's installation manual.
•4. Place system in accordance with laser system specifications.
•5. Post caution signs.
•6. Install cavity components on rail as recommended by installation manual.

9.2.2 Water Lines

•1. Test water temperature to see that it is in specified range indicated in service manual. If water temperature is too high, increase flow or install an external chiller.
•2. Connect input and output secondary water lines to heat exchanger.
•3. Connect input and output primary (closed loop) water lines to laser head.
•4. Fill cooler reservoir with deionized water.
•5. Turn on cooler switch.
•6. Check that water is circulating through head.

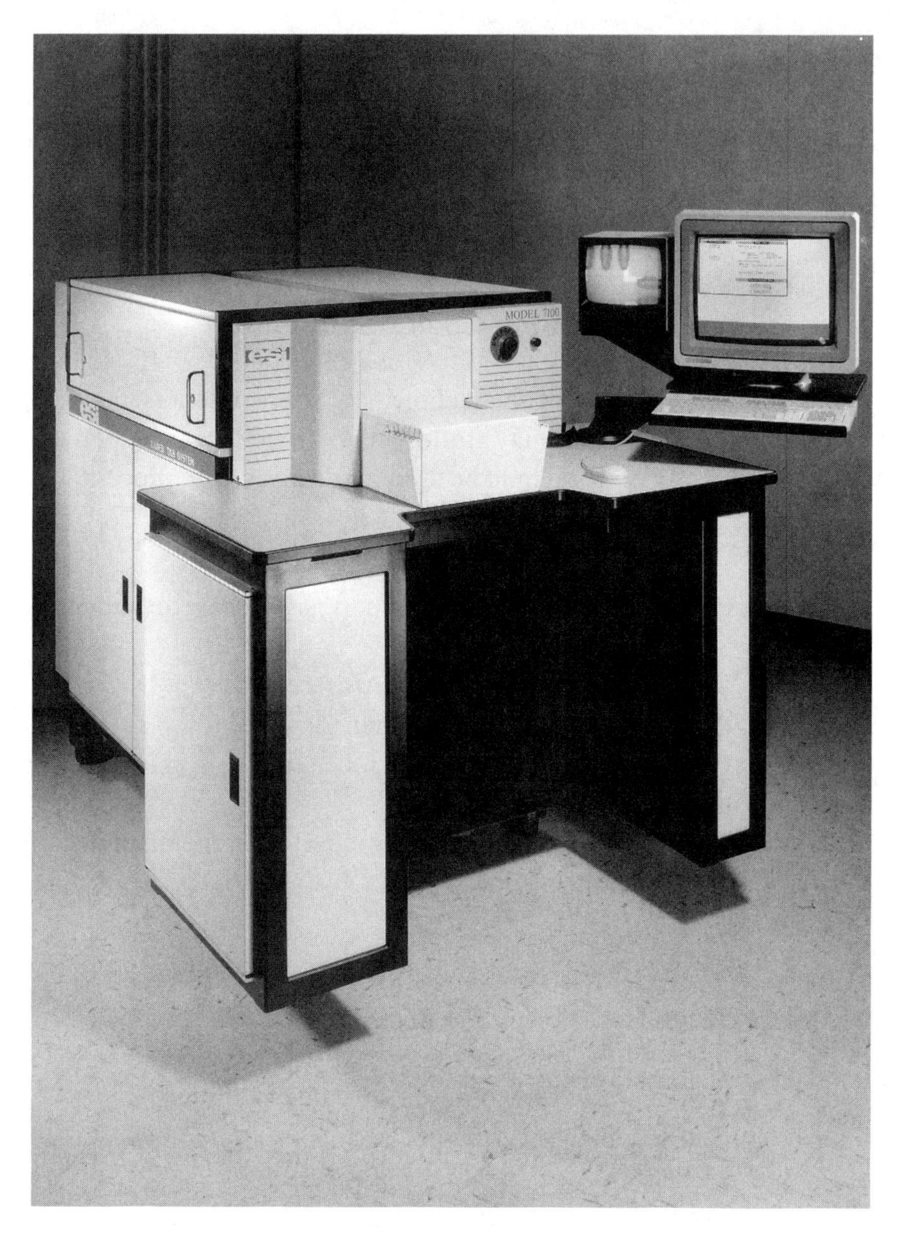

Figure 9-18 Typical Nd:YAG system
(*Courtesy of Electro Scientific Industries, Inc.*)

9.2.3 Electrical Power

(CAUTION: PROCEED WITH ALL POWER OFF)

•1. Connect laser high voltage connector from power supply to laser head.
•2. Connect interlock cable from RF driver to laser head.
•3. Connect RF BNC cable from RF driver to laser head.
•4. Connect input voltage power cable to laser power supply.
•5. Inspect system and correct for loose or broken connections before applying power.
•6. Plug voltage input cable into voltage source.

9.2.4 Start-Up Operation

•1. Review safety policies and procedures.
•2. Remove obstacles from beam path.
•3. Place beam stop at end of beam path.
•4. Put on safety goggles.
•5. Energize laser according to manufacturer's instructions.
•6. Note that lamp fires.
•7. Set current to recommended range according to service manual.
•8. Place black light and phosphor screen in front of beam expander.
•9. Open shutter.
•10. Observe that laser is operating by viewing phosphor screen.
•11. Measure output beam power using meter and record.

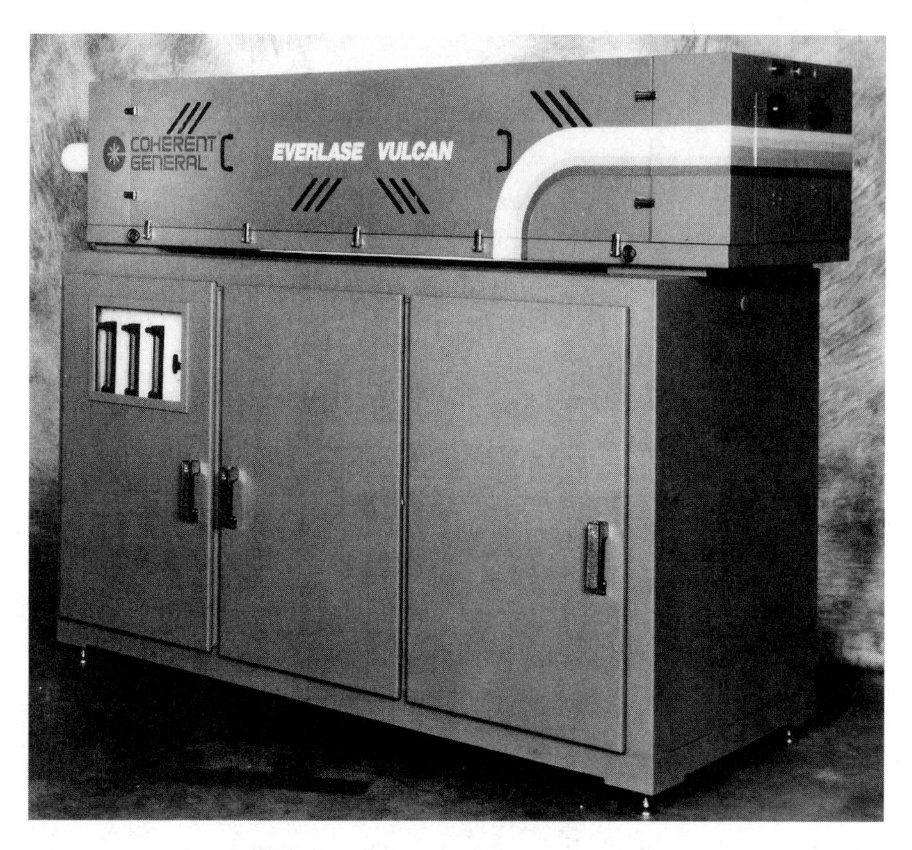

Figure 9-19 Complete CO_2 laser system
(Courtesy of Coherent General, Inc.)

9.3 Installing a Gas Discharge Laser

Information in this section is given in a step-by-step form so that the reader may follow the procedure sequentially. Manufacturer's guidelines should be used for details on the process.

9.3.1 Inspection

- •1. Unpack crates and verify parts with inventory or packing slip.
- •2. Read manufacturer's installation manual.
- •3. Place laser system in accordance with specifications.
- •4. Post caution signs.
- •5. Put on safety goggles.
- •6. Level laser head according to installation manual.
- •7. Tie down laser as suggested.
- •8. Align laser cavity with HeNe alignment laser.

9.3.2 Water Lines

- •1. Test water temperature to see that it is in specified range indicated in service manual. If water temperature is too high, increase flow or install an external chiller.
- •2. Connect input and output secondary water lines to heat exchanger.
- •3. Connect input and output primary (closed loop) water lines to laser head.
- •4. Turn on cooler switch.
- •5. Check that water is circulating through head.

9.3.3 Electrical Power

(CAUTION: PROCEED WITH ALL POWER OFF)

- •1. Connect laser high voltage connector from power supply to laser head.
- •2. Connect input voltage power cable to laser power supply.

•3. Inspect system and correct for loose or broken connections before applying power.
•4. Plug voltage input cable into voltage source.

9.3.3 Gas Supply

•1. Connect gas to flow control unit.
•2. Connect flow control to laser head.

9.3.4 Start-Up Operation

•1. Review safety policies and procedures.
•2. Remove obstacles from beam path.
•3. Place beam stop at end of beam path.
•4. Put on safety goggles.
•5. Energize laser according to manufacturer's instructions.
•6. Note that laser tube fires.
•7. Set current to recommended range according to service manual.
•8. Place black light and phosphor screen in front of beam expander.
•9. Open shutter.
•10. Observe that laser is operating by viewing phosphor screen.
•11. Measure output beam power using meter and record.

10

MEDIUM POWER LASERS

Introduction

Lasers with output powers below one kilowatt, but still above the milliwatt levels of smaller lasers, can be described as medium-power lasers. Argon, ruby, and krypton lasers are common examples. These lasers are not nearly as large, and in certain ways not nearly as complex, as the Nd:YAG or CO_2 lasers discussed in the previous chapter—but they do require some maintenance and repair.

Since some of the problems (and their accompanying solutions) encountered with medium-power lasers are very similar to the high-power lasers, Chapter 10 will not provide as much detail in troubleshooting, and the reader might refer to Chapter 9 for more revealing discussions. However, because medium-power laser beams are less formidable (lower power and generally visible wavelengths), they do allow for more in the way of beam diagnostics. Consequently, these will be discussed in detail. Such diagnostic methods also apply, in general, to the low-power lasers of the next chapter.

10.1 Troubleshooting Guide

In troubleshooting, the argon laser and the ruby laser will be used as common examples for medium-power lasers. The information on troubleshooting is provided in a flowchart format so the reader may quickly locate the problem, its possible causes, and the likely solutions.

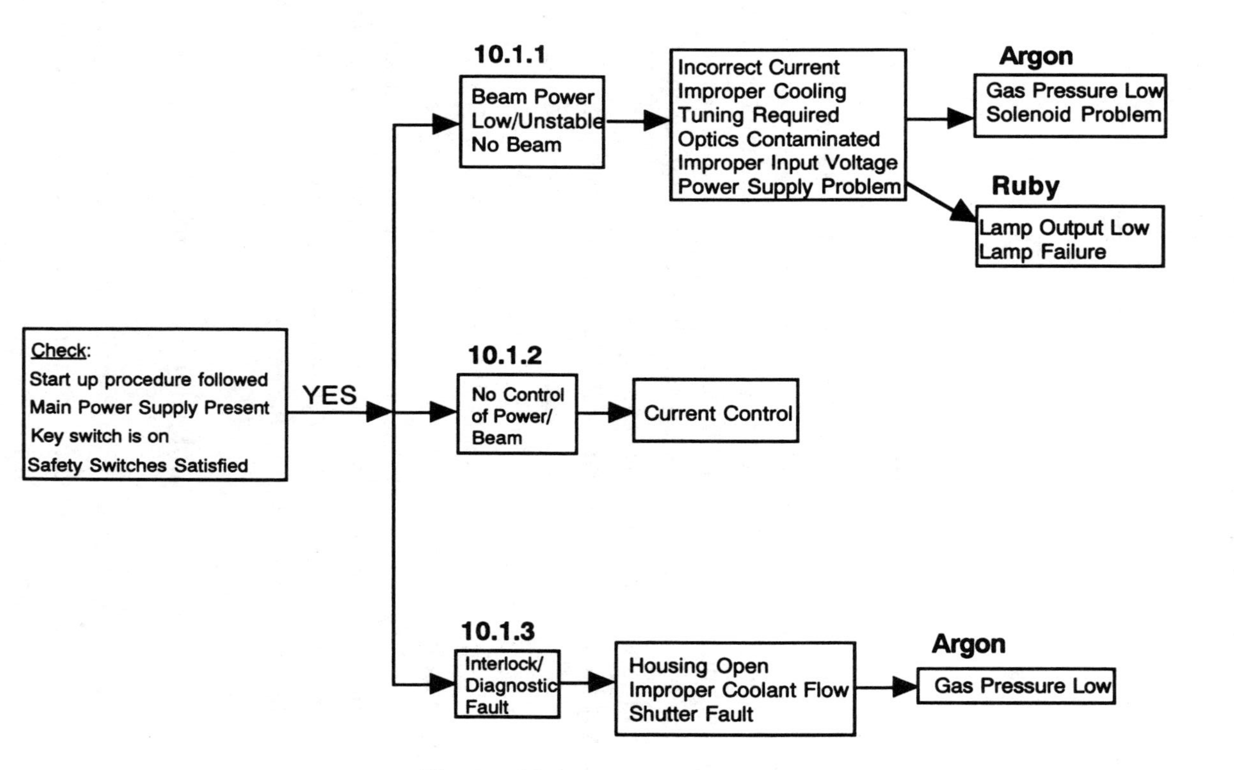

Figure 10-1 Troubleshooting Flowchart

The elements of the flow chart are discussed in the pages that follow it. As with high-power lasers, it is strongly suggested that manufacturer's guidelines be followed whenever possible. The information in this section is meant as a general guide and should not take precedence over manufacturer's suggestions.

10.1.1 Beam Power Low or Unstable, No Beam

If proper startup procedures are followed and the laser refuses to fire or the beam is erratic, the problem may be one of several. The current must be set to a proper level for the gas to ionize in an argon laser, and for the lamp to fire in a ruby laser. Improper cooling, contaminated or misaligned optics, and problems with supply voltage will also lead to beam problems. In the case of an argon laser, low gas pressure will affect the beam, and a failure of the flash lamp will lead to problems for the ruby laser.

Incorrect Current. The current control for the laser has a minimum setting that can be used for startup. If the current is set below this minimum, the power supply will be unable to ionize the gas and produce a beam. Current is usually measured and displayed by a built-in meter, and the meter reading should be compared to manufacturer's suggestions for startup current. The startup current may be smaller than the minimum current required to operate the laser once lasing begins.

Improper Cooling. Cooling for medium-power lasers is usually accomplished by pumping water around the cavity (and the lamp in a solid laser). If the flow of the water is too slow, or if the temperature of the incoming water is too high, the laser will not be cooled enough to fire. Improper cooling can also lead to unstable or low beam power.

The schematic diagram of a cooling circuit is shown in Figure 10-2. The shutoff valves should be checked to make sure they are open. Most medium-power lasers make use of a continuous flow of water rather than a temperature regulated control. If your laser allows the water to flow continuously, check the lines to see if water is flowing through them (water can usually be felt or heard as it moves through the line). Also, inspect lines for cracks, leaks, or other signs of wear.

Lasers with a flow control device may have a faulty temperature sensor or valve. In addition to the checks listed above, these two devices should be inspected. Even though such valves are electronically controlled, it is usually possible to manually open and close them to verify that they are operating correctly.

Tuning Required. Mirror alignment is critical to the laser's operation. Over time, laser mirrors may fall out of alignment and cause problems in the beam. If the mirrors are misaligned, the beam power will be less than normal, and misalignment may even lead to no beam at all.

Manufacturer's guidelines for tuning the cavity should be followed. In general, tuning is a two-step process that begins with a rough adjustment using an autocollimator or the beam from a low power laser. Fine adjustments can be made by tweaking the adjustment screws on the laser while monitoring the output power. Great care should be exercised while performing the second step since it involves overriding the interlocks of the laser and operating it while the cavity is exposed. Extreme hazards exist from high voltage and from the beam itself. Safety goggles should be worn at all times, and standard high voltage safety practices followed. Cavity tuning should not be attempted by an untrained person.

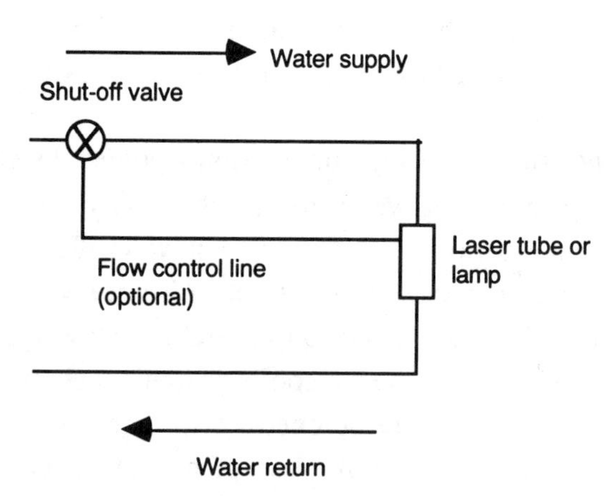

Figure 10-2 Schematic of a cooling circuit

Some smaller lasers have sealed cavities that do not allow for adjusting the mirrors. These cavities are easy to identify since the mirror mounts will not have adjustment screws, and, in the case of gas lasers, the mirrors will be affixed directly to the tube. Such lasers do not require tuning since the mirrors are permanently fixed in position. Figure 10-3 illustrates the tunable and the sealed cavity.

The diagram is a schematic representation and does not show many of the parts of the cavity that are normally present.

Optics Contaminated. The surfaces of the optics in lasers that are not sealed are subject to contamination from dust and to damage if they are not handled properly. These changes to the surface of the optics will result in a loss of power and in a degradation of beam quality. Dirty optics can be cleaned following manufacturer's guidelines, although great care should be taken. The optics are highly sensitive and proper procedures and materials should be used. Cleaning usually involves removing particles by blowing the optics with clean air (standard compressed air should never be used) or by brushing with a fine, camel's hair brush. The surfaces should then be wiped using a lens tissue and a lens cleaning solution (methanol or acetone are possible cleaners but should not be used on plastic optics or on optics with certain coatings). The cleaner is applied to the surface of the optical component or to the lens tissue, and then the tissue is dragged slowly across the surface without applying any pressure. A clean tissue should be used for each pass.

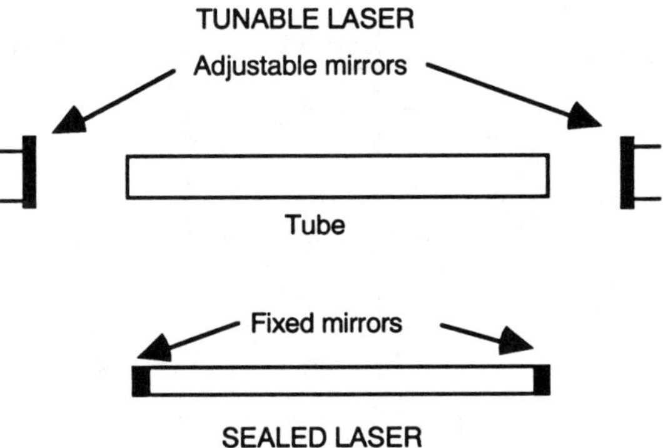

Figure 10-3 Tunable and Sealed Lasers
(Parts of the cavity are not pictured)

Improper Input Voltage. The input voltage to the laser's power supply should meet certain standards set by the manufacturer. The voltage for medium-power lasers may be single phase or three phase and is often 208 or 240 volts. If this input voltage is not correct, the power supply will not output the proper voltage to the laser head.

Fluctuations in the service to the building that houses the laser may affect input voltages, and the input voltage should be checked if a problem occurs. Standard input voltages can usually be measured with a VOM (volt-ohm-milliameter) or a digital meter. Care should be taken when measuring the voltages because shock hazards exist.

Power Supply Problem. If the power supply is not operating properly, the laser cavity will not receive the proper voltage and current to operate correctly, which will lead to fluctuations in beam power and possibly no beam at all.

Power supplies for medium power lasers generally consist of a step-up transformer, a voltage multiplier circuit, and a rectifier. Often a second circuit provides a high voltage trigger pulse to ionize the gas before operation. If the laser is pulsed, it may have a circuit pulsing the power supply output. Figure 10-4 illustrates a common power supply circuit for a solid laser.

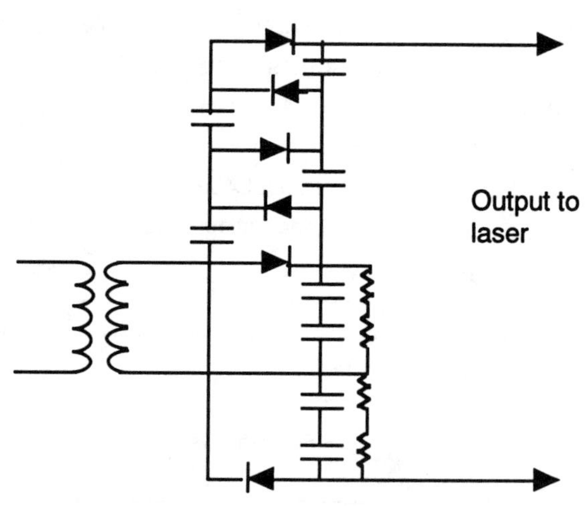

Figure 10-4 Power supply

Problems with power supplies fall into the field of electronics. Section 9.1.2 in Chapter 9 offers some suggestions about checking the individual components in the circuit. In general, the power supply output can be checked with a high voltage probe, but caution should be exercised when dealing with such high voltage values. The probe should be connected with the high voltage turned off. The reading should be made without touching the probe or the meter when the high voltage is turned on. If the output of the supply is not correct, check fuses in the circuit as well as the input voltage.

Argon Lasers—Gas Pressure. The gas pressure in an argon laser is critical to its proper operation. Larger lasers have a system for adding gas to the tube and are equipped with a gauge that indicates the pressure. Manufacturer's suggestions on gas pressure should be followed, but it is important to realize that the gas pressure will be lower when the laser is first turned on than it will be once the laser has been operating for a while and has a chance to heat up. Do not add gas to a "cold" laser without first checking the manufacturer's suggestions about startup pressures.

Sealed argon lasers do not allow for adding gas to the cavity, and when the pressure starts to change, only replacement of the tube can rectify the problem. Fortunately, the laser will generally operate at lower pressures even though the output power will be lower.

Argon Lasers—Solenoid Problem. Argon lasers incorporate a coil that produces a magnetic field in the cavity (see Chapter 2). If this coil is not operating correctly, output power will be reduced. The coil generally has a separate supply voltage from the power supply and this voltage should be measured and compared to the manufacturer's suggested voltage (often labeled on the power supply). If the voltage is too low, the power supply is at fault.

The coil itself can be checked by measuring its resistance. An infinitely large resistance indicates an opening in the coil. Resistances smaller than indicated by the laser manual indicate the coil is shorted somewhere.

Ruby Lasers—Low Lamp Output. Over time, the flash lamp or arc lamp used in ruby and other solid lasers will degenerate. The output power of these lamps will be smaller due to deposits on the surface of the lamp caused by eroding electrodes and sputter (due to operating at low currents). The lamp can be examined for deposits that appear as a white, grainy substance on the inside of the lamp (for electrode erosion) and as black spots from sputter. The amount of deposit will govern how much the lamp power has declined.

Lamps are rated in terms of hours of operation (or in terms of shots for flash lamps) and the manufacturer will indicate how frequently a lamp should be replaced. Advanced decay of the lamp may even lead to zero output from the laser.

Ruby Lasers—Lamp Failure. Lamps may fail in one of two ways. Over a prolonged period of time, the deposits described above will reach a point where the lamp is no longer able to provide enough light to operate the laser.

A catastrophic failure (lamp explodes) may occur from operation at current values that are too high or from increasing the current too rapidly. Lamps have a polarity (anode and cathode) and if they are connected backwards, they will explode. In addition, some lamps may be "rogue" lamps, which fail because of improper construction.

10.1.2 No Control of Beam Power

Beam power is controlled by adjusting the current supplied to the laser. If the current control circuitry is faulty, beam power control will not respond. Current control is often accomplished by means of a variac (or adjustable transformer) which controls the input voltage to the power supply. More complex power supplies may control current using power transistors or similar components. Troubleshooting these components is a general electronics problem, and is beyond the scope of this book. Manufacturer's suggestions for checking the current control should be followed.

10.1.3 Interlock Fault

Lasers are equipped with interlocks which monitor certain parts of the laser and shut down operation or provide warning signals if a fault occurs. Interlocks may be wired to separate indicators so the problem can be pinpointed, or they may be connected to a general interlock fault indicator. Some common sense should be exercised when locating the cause of an interlock fault since there may be more than one possible problem that leads to the fault. For example, a cooling fault may be simply the result of a valve being closed, and not a general problem with the cooling circuitry.

Housing. The housing that covers the laser cavity and the power supply is equipped with an interlock that prevents the laser from operating if the housing is removed or opened. This prevents accidental exposure to high voltage and hazardous light emissions. Sometimes it's necessary to operate the laser with a housing open, in which case the interlock has to be defeated. Great care should be exercised when operating a laser with the interlock defeated since hazards from high voltage, the beam, and the lamp are present. Safety goggles should be worn at all times.

Cooling. Some lasers monitor the temperature of the cavity and the temperature and flow of the coolant, and will shut down the laser if improper levels are reached. The cooling system should be checked as described in section 10.1.1.

Shutter Fault. Shutters in the laser prevent output of the beam when it is not required. Some shutters are equipped with indicators that show when the shutter is open. Medium-power laser shutters are not as complex as those used in high-power lasers, and they are not usually equipped with fault devices that will shut down the laser if the shutter fails.

Argon Lasers—Gas Pressure. Larger argon lasers have devices that monitor gas pressure and will indicate when gas pressure is too low. Some lasers have indicator lights while others emit a high-pitched tone.

The gas pressure should be kept at manufacturer's specifications (see section 10.1.1).

10.2 Beam Diagnostics

Often it is necessary to check the properties of the laser beam to make sure they match what is required or specified. Beam diagnostics include: checking beam power or energy; beam divergence and profile; pulse characteristics; and wavelength and bandwidth.

The principles of calibration and traceability in beam diagnostics are very important for medical lasers, which must be precisely controlled and well documented. There are currently no complete standards for beam diagnostics, although some calibration standards for power and energy are provided by certain agencies.

10.2.1 Near Field, Far Field, and Beam Waist

When measuring spatial properties of laser beam, it is important to note that *where* the measurements are made is important. A Gaussian laser beam (see below) is always diverging away from some point, or converging toward some point. This point represents the minimum diameter, known as the beam waist, and is shown in Figure 10-5. Close to the beam waist is an area known as the *near field* of the beam, where divergence and diameter are not constant. At large distances from the beam waist is the *far field* where measurements are normally made. Measurements made in the near field will not be consistent with those made in the far field. The far field of a laser beam is the area where most laser applications occur. In the absence of any external optics, the beam waist of a laser can be assumed to be at the output mirror.

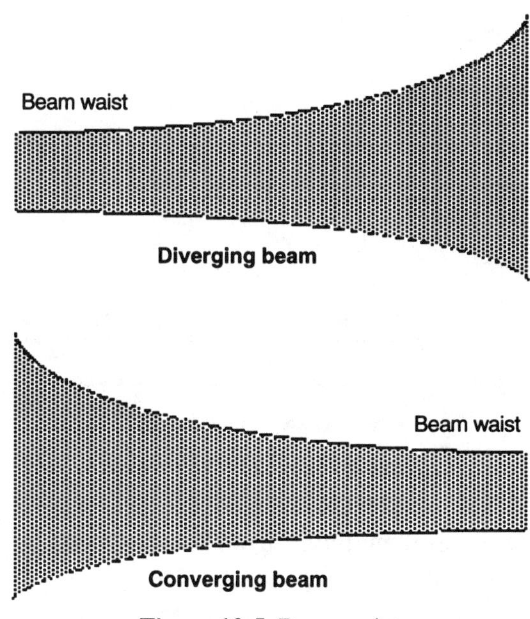

Figure 10-5 Beam waist

10.2.2 Measuring Beam Diameter

Beam diameters' discussions and measurements are usually confined to Gaussian beam distributions (see Chapter 1). The profile of a laser that outputs in the TEM_{00} mode has the shape illustrated in Figure 10-6 and is known as a Gaussian beam, since the Gaussian profile changes its width at different points, but the beam diameter is defined as the width of this profile at the point where the power is equal to the maximum power divided by e^2. This is not a random point, but one that fits in with the mathematics used to describe the Gaussian beam.

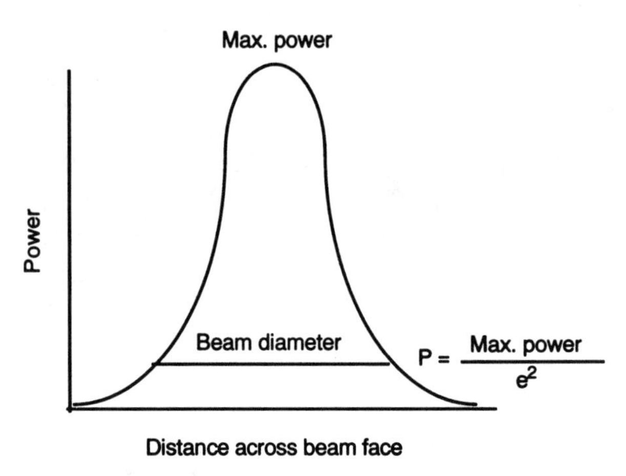

Figure 10-6 Gaussian profile

There are several methods used to measure the diameter of a Gaussian beam, and they vary in terms of complexity, sophistication, and precision. Advanced beam diagnostic equipment, such as the Coherent Lab Master® allows a technician to illuminate a detector with the beam and then provide a detailed readout of the beam's properties. These systems use electronically scanned detectors and sophisticated circuitry to provide the information and are the ideal method for diagnosing the beam. However, limited resources and cost often require using some of the less-sophisticated methods that are described below.

Aperture Transmission. The diameter of a laser beam can be roughly determined by passing it through an aperture of a known size that is smaller than the beam itself. Since the aperture will block a percentage of the beam in proportion to the beam's diameter and the aperture's diameter, it is possible to calculate the beam diameter by measuring the amount that is blocked. The experimental setup is illustrated in Figure 10-7. The beam is passed through the aperture and the power is measured before (P_{before}) the aperture and after the aperture (P_{after}). The fraction of the light transmitted by the aperture (T) is calculated by

$$T = P_{after} / P_{before} \qquad \text{(Equation 10.1)}$$

The diameter of the beam (Z) can be calculated using the diameter of the aperture (a) and the fraction of light transmitted (T) in Equation 10.2.

$$Z = \text{sq. rt.} \left((2a^2) / \ln(1/(1-T))\right) \quad \text{(Equation 10.2)}$$

The aperture transmission method is not extremely precise, but it does offer a simple method (that does not require expensive equipment) for measuring beam diameter.

Mechanical Scanning. To make a more precise measurement of beam diameter, a detector can be mounted on a linear translator or similar device that allows precise linear movement. The detector is then moved across the face of the beam — power readings and detector positions are recorded at several intervals. This scanning method is illustrated in Figure 10-8, and the resulting data are then plotted to produce a curve similar to the one shown in Figure 10-6. The diameter of the laser beam is determined by finding the point where the power equals the maximum divided by e^2 and noting the width of the curve at that point.

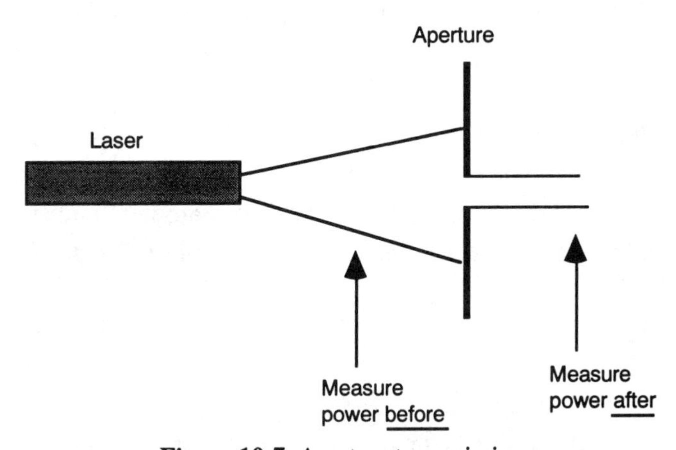

Figure 10-7 Aperture transmission

It is important that the light sensitive area of the detector be smaller than the beam. Otherwise, the resulting curve will have a flattened shape because the detector will provide a maximum reading at several points. If the detector area is larger than the beam, the width of the detector will have to be factored out of the resulting data before a realistic diameter can be calculated.

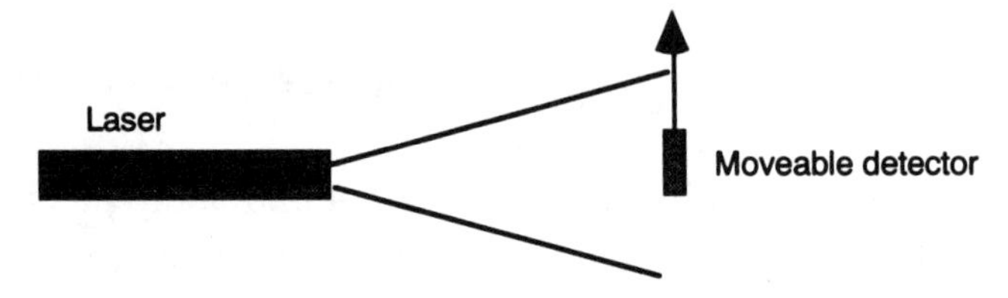

Record power and position at several points along the face of the beam.

Figure 10-8 Scanning method

10.2.3 Measuring Beam Divergence

The diameter of the laser beam is continuously changing as a result of divergence (see Chapter 1). Since the laser is always diverging or converging, its diameter constantly increases or decreases. Measuring the change in beam diameter, or the beam divergence, is as important as measuring the diameter itself. Divergence allows prediction of diameter at a given point and is also a factor in focusing the laser beam (see Chapter 6).

Two Diameter Method. The beam divergence can be calculated by measuring the diameter at two different distances from the laser. The divergence (θ) is calculated by using the two diameters and the distance from the laser at the two different points, as shown in Equation 10.3.

$$\theta = (d_1 - d_2)/(l_1 - l_2) \qquad \text{(Equation 10.3)}$$

where

d_1 and d_2 = the diameters at the two points, and
l_1 and l_2 = the distances from the laser.

Focusing Lens Method. By using a focusing, or converging, lens, the beam divergence can be calculated with only one diameter measurement. Since the beam divergence, diameter, and the lens's focal length are related (see Chapter 6), the divergence can be measured as shown in

Figure 10-9. The lens should have a focal length that is at least ten times the beam diameter and should be placed at a distance from the laser which is much less than the Raleigh range (z_r) given by

$$z_r = \pi d^2/r\lambda \qquad \text{(Equation 10.4)}$$

where

d = beam diameter, and
λ = the laser beam wavelength.

The beam diameter is measured at the focal point of the lens and divergence is calculated by

$$\theta = d/f \qquad \text{(Equation 10.5)}$$

where

f = focal length of the lens.

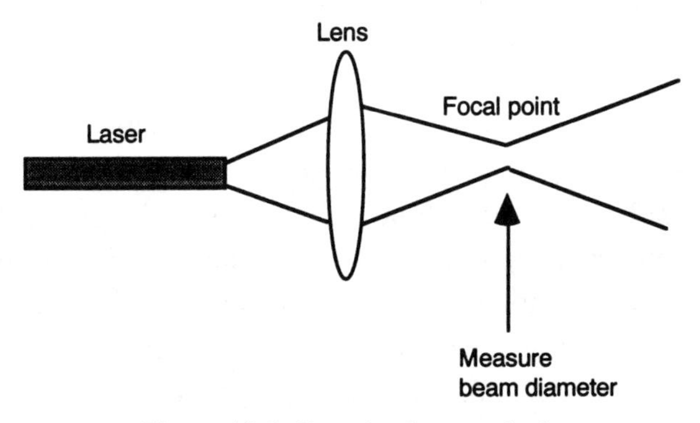

Figure 10-9 Focusing lens method

10.2.4 Measuring Wavelength

The output of many lasers can contain several wavelengths; many applications require a precise determination of the wavelength and the bandwidth (or spread of wavelengths) of the beam. Measuring wavelength can be accomplished using a device known as a monochromator. Etalons (see Chapter 3) can also be used to measure wavelength.

Monochromators. A monochromator is a standard device for measuring wavelength. The monochromator incorporates an optical component such as a diffraction grating or a prism (see Chapter 3) that separates light by wavelength. The light that enters the monochromator is split into several rays, each of which is a separate wavelength and is traveling in a different direction. Figure 10-10 shows a simple monochromator that makes use of a diffraction grating.

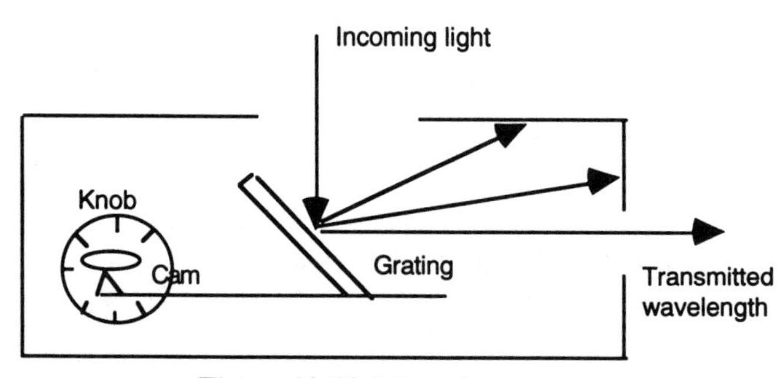

Figure 10-10 Monochromator

Light entering the monochromator is reflected from the grating and split into separate rays. The grating is rotated by means of a calibrated knob and a cam. Since different wavelengths will reflect at different angles, adjusting the knob will allow specific wavelengths to pass out of the monochromator. The knob can be set to specific wavelengths, and a laser beam passing into the monochromator will only be emitted if its wavelength is the same as the monochromator's setting.

Monochromators are useful devices for measuring laser beams that have several, well-spaced wavelengths (such as tunable dye lasers). A detector may be placed at the output aperture and used to pinpoint the wavelengths present in the beam. For more precise measurements, such as determining the longitudinal modes of a beam (see Chapter 1), the optical element in the monochromator may not have enough resolution to do the job. In such cases, an etalon arrangement is used.

Etalon Scanning. An etalon consists of two reflecting surfaces that are flat, and perpendicular to each other. The surfaces are separated and the material between them may be air or may be the same as the surface material. When light is incident on one surface of the etalon (see Figure 10-11), it is split into multiple parts by reflection and refraction.

The separated rays will undergo the same process at the second surface and a fraction of the light will emerge from the opposite side of the etalon. The light that passes through the etalon will experience a phase shift due to differences in path length and due to the reflections. For a given distance between the two surfaces, only one wavelength of light will emerge from the etalon in phase. Other wavelengths will be out of phase and will experience destructive interference (for more on phase and interference see Chapter 1 section 1.2.2 and Chapter 8 section 8.1). Because of this phase effect, the etalon will transmit specific wavelengths depending on the distance between the two surfaces. If the distance between the mirrors is adjustable, the etalon can be used to measure the wavelengths in a laser beam, as well as identify the longitudinal modes and their separation.

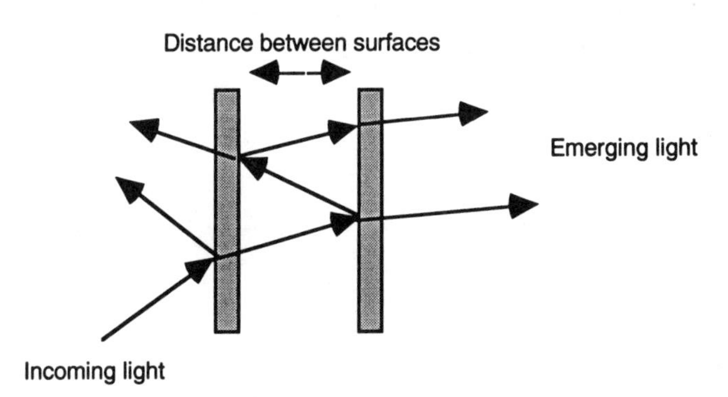

Figure 10-11 Etalon

The laser outputs several longitudinal modes which depend on wavelength, cavity size and shape, and gain. Identifying these modes and their separation is an important part of beam diagnostics. The setup for detecting and measuring longitudinal modes, their width and their separation is shown in Figure 10-12. The laser beam passes through the etalon and is incident on a detector. The output of the detector is shown on the oscilloscope display. For different wavelengths (and different modes) the scope will show different peak voltage values. When the etalon is adjusted for a wavelength present in the beam, the scope will indicate a voltage peak at a certain point on the time scale.

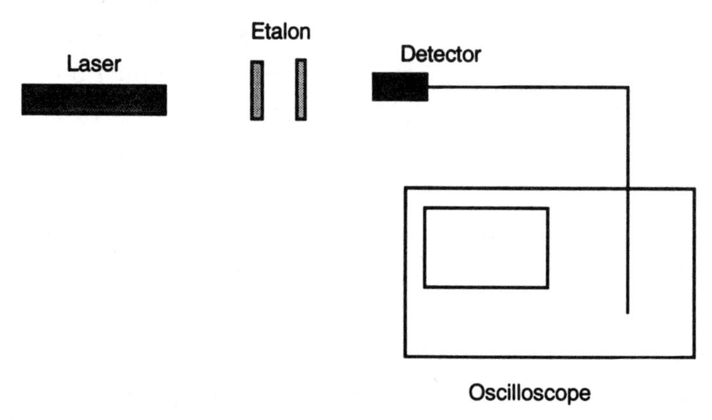

Figure 10-12 Measuring longitudinal modes

When the etalon is adjusted for a new wavelength, the peak will occur at a different position on the time scale. The height of the peak will provide information about the power of the mode, and the position of the peak will provide information about the separation between the modes. Finally, the width of the peaks corresponds to the width of the mode.

BIBLIOGRAPHY

Laser/Electro-Optic Measurements–Course X. Waco, TX: Center for Occupational Research and Development, 1985.

Laser Technology. Waco, TX: Center for Occupational Research and Development, 1985.

O'Shea, Donald. *Elements of Modern Optical Design.* New York: John Wiley & Sons, Inc., 1985.

11

LOW-POWER LASERS

Introduction

Low-power lasers, such as the helium neon and the semiconductor, represent some unique challenges for the laser technician. Repair and troubleshooting are limited (especially in the case of the semiconductor laser) and are generally electronic in nature. The helium neon laser is generally composed of a tube with sealed and fixed mirrors and a printed circuit board that contains the power supply. Any repair work that might be performed is limited to this circuit board. Since troubleshooting circuit boards and electronic components is somewhat beyond the scope of this book, discussion of helium neon lasers will be limited to a few practical suggestions and observations.

However, the semiconductor laser requires some particular procedures in handling, operation, and basic setup. These procedures are essential for anyone who does any significant work with this laser type. It should be noted that it is possible to purchase semiconductor lasers in self-contained packages that eliminate most of the work discussed in this chapter. These packaged lasers require little more than an external D.C. voltage source (often a battery or combination of batteries will suffice); they are limited, however, in terms of the range and usefulness of their applications.

11.1 Semiconductor Lasers

Semiconductor lasers are sensitive to many outside forces. The output of the laser changes significantly with drive current and temperature. The laser can be destroyed by transients cause by static electricity and voltage or current spikes from the operating supply. Light reflected into the laser cavity can also cause problems.

To guard against damage and to ensure proper operation, semiconductor lasers must be properly handled, mounted, and equipped with external devices and circuitry. Care and setup can be classified into four broad areas of interest—temperature sensitivity, current sensitivity, protection against static electricity, and optical feedback sensitivity.

11.1.1 Temperature Sensitivity

The output of a semiconductor laser is greatly affected by its temperature. Increases in temperature will cause decreases in the output power of the laser and increases in threshold current (see section 11.1.2). In addition, changes in temperature cause changes in the spectral content of the beam. Various measures are used to limit the change in temperature of the laser and minimize these effects.

Figure 11-1 illustrates the effects of temperature on the output power of the laser. Temperature T1 is the lowest and temperature T3 is the highest. Notice that as the temperature increases, the laser requires additional current to sustain the same output power. Increasing current leads to a vicious circle since its additional current leads to increased temperature. Figure 11-1 also shows that the threshold current (minimum current required to produce a laser beam) increases with temperature.

Spectral content of the beam also changes with temperature, as shown in Figure 11-2. The peak (or main) output wavelength will shift as the temperature increases. Figure 11-2 likewise shows that mode structure of the beam changes. The number of modes, their intensity, and even their separation can change. To compensate for these fluctuations, the laser must be kept at a reasonably low and, more importantly, stable temperature. Temperature control is accomplished through the use of heat sinks or feedback and cooling circuitry. Applications which do not require specific wavelengths (such as alignment and pointing) do not require most of the precautions discussed below.

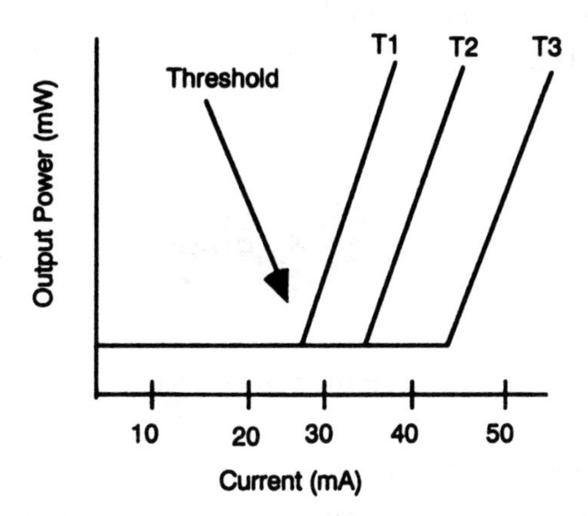

Figure 11-1 Output power as a function of temperature (graph is an illustration and is not meant to represent actual data)

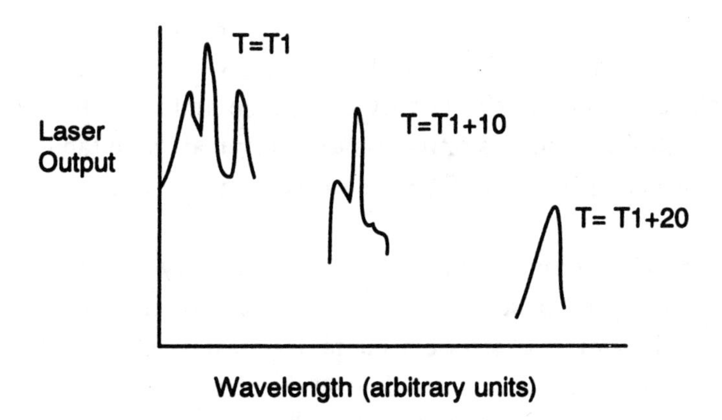

Figure 11-2 Beam output at three separate temperatures (graph is an illustration and is not meant to represent actual data)

Heat Sinks. A heat sink is a thermally conductive plate that is mounted on the laser (see Figure 11-3). The heat sink has several fins cut into it which are designed to remove excess heat from the laser and radiate it to the surrounding air. The heat sink is the first stage of temperature control and its size and shape are designed to remove a substantial amount of heat. Often, heat sinks are used with heat sink compound, a paste that increases the thermal conductivity and helps draw the heat away from the laser.

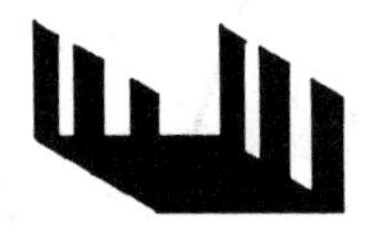

Figure 11-3 Heat sink

Feedback Circuitry. To maintain a stable temperature, the laser must be equipped with circuitry to monitor the temperature and cool the laser. One possible solution is to mount a thermistor (temperature dependent resistor) in close proximity to the laser and with good thermal connection to it. The thermistor is incorporated into a wheatstone bridge arrangement which is in turn connected to a thermoelectric cooler (or a Peltier element). When the laser increases in temperature, the thermistor changes resistance and the bridge is thrown out of balance. The thermoelectric cooler is driven by the bridge and accompanies to cool the laser until the thermistor returns to its original value (and the laser to its original temperature). This feedback circuit is illustrated in Figure 11-4.

The electronics of the circuit are relatively simple since a few resistors, an operational amplifier, and the thermal circuits are all that are required. However, careful consideration must be given to the thermal loads and mass as well as the delays in the circuitry. In general, a basic circuit is created and tested and then components are changed to compensate for these problems. For precise applications, it is often important to maintain temperature within less than one degree.

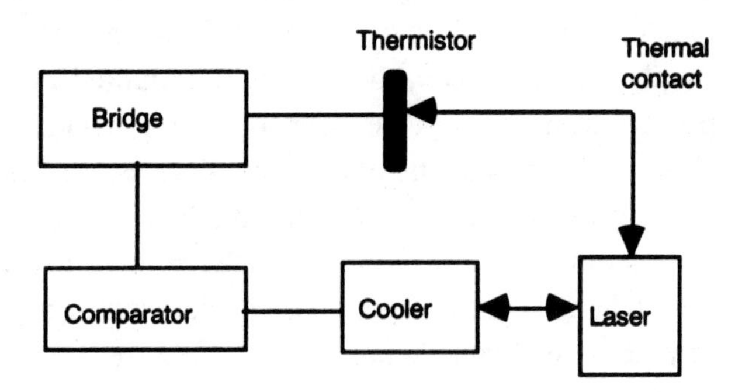

Figure 11-4 Cooling circuitry

11.1.2 Current Sensitivity

The drive current of the semiconductor laser, like the temperature, affects the output. Semiconductor lasers have a minimum current required for operation (known as the threshold current). Beyond this minimum, output power increases with drive current as shown in Figure 11-5. The semiconductor laser also has a maximum current beyond which the laser will be damaged or destroyed. Increasing the current not only increases the output power, it also changes the output wavelength. The wavelength will shift with increased current and the number and shape of the modes will change (see Figure 11-5) in much the same way as with an increase in temperature.

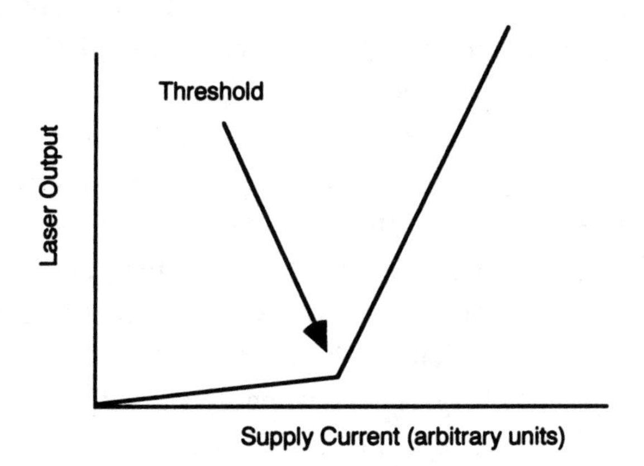

Figure 11-5 Threshold current

To protect against these shifts due to current, the power supply for semiconductor lasers must be well regulated and the laser equipped with a monitor photodiode. The photodiode is mounted at one end of the laser (opposite from the end used for the output beam) and, since light escapes from both ends of the cavity, the diode can be used to measure the output power of the laser. The photodiode is connected to the power supply and its output is used to regulate the amount of current supplied to the laser. Changes in the output beam will result in adjustments in the current by this feedback arrangement. Figure 11-6 illustrates the monitor photodiode and its operation.

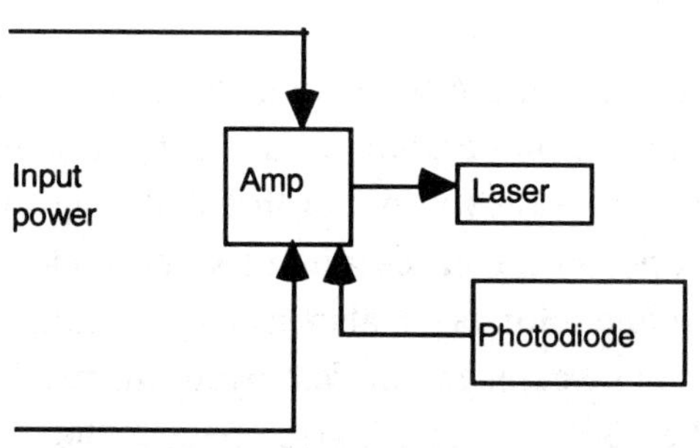

Figure 11-6 Monitor photodiode

11.1.3 Protection Against Static Electricity

The semiconductor laser can be easily damaged by transients caused by static electricity discharging through the laser. To protect against this, standard practices for static electricity sensitive components must be followed. The two areas of importance are grounding and shielding. To prevent a buildup of static electricity on the body, technicians working with semiconductor lasers should be properly grounded. Grounding is generally accomplished by wearing a grounding strap that is attached to the wrist and to an appropriate ground. In addition to the technician, the bench or table that is used for the work-place should also be grounded or equipped with a rubber mat to protect against static electricity. The laser itself should be packaged and stored in conductive foam or in conductive plastic containers which are designed for static electricity sensitive components. Once in operation, the laser should be protected against electrical hazards by housing it in a metallic case which is properly grounded and which will shield it.

11.1.4 Optical Feedback

When the beam of the semiconductor laser is incident on a reflective surface (such as lenses or even lightly colored walls and mounts) there is a possibility that some of the beam will be scattered back into the laser cavity. This optical feedback will lead to problems in laser operation. Stray light re-entering the cavity will cause shifts in the output wavelength and variations in the output power. This effect is present in all lasers, but it is especially worrisome in a semiconductor laser since the results are much more noticeable.

To prevent unwanted light from re-entering the laser cavity, an isolator must be used. The isolator is based on the principles of polarization (see Chapter 3) and allows light of only one polarization to pass through it. By placing a polarizer in front of the laser and before any optics or other objects, the reflected light will be stopped, since the emitted beam will undergo a change in polarization due to the reflection. Optical feedback is especially a concern when optics are mounted close to the laser cavity.

11.2 Helium Neon Lasers

As mentioned in the introduction, helium neon lasers do not offer much opportunity for troubleshooting beyond repairing the power supply. Since it is generally sealed and the mirrors fixed, the helium neon laser cavity is virtually non repairable. Fortunately, the cost of helium neon lasers is relatively low and replacing the laser is not normally difficult.

There are some practical tips about helium neon lasers that will help to extend their operating life and allow for some simple repair. In terms of operation, the helium neon laser, as a gas discharge device, will last longer and operate better when it is left on for an extended period of time. Continuous operation over a few hours is much more beneficial to the laser than repeatedly turning the laser off and on. In fact, if the laser is not used very often, manufacturers often recommend operating the laser for a few hours each month to extend the lifetime of the tube.

The output of the helium neon will gradually lose power as the laser increases in age. Often the loss in power is not enough to make the laser useless unless the application requires a certain minimum power level. When the laser loses too much power (or ceases to operate completely) it is possible to purchase the tube separately from the power supply so that the replacement cost is reduced.

BIBLIOGRAPHY

Laser Technology. Waco, TX: Center for Occupational Research and Development, 1985.

Wieman, Carl and Holberg, Leo. "Using Diode Lasers for Atomic Physics" *Science Instrumentation*, Vol. 62, No. 1, January 1991.

Appendix A

USEFUL CONSTANTS AND PHYSICAL DATA

Table 1 Useful Constants and Physical Data	
Speed of Light (vacuum)	2.998×10^{8} m/s
Planck's Constant	6.6×10^{-34} j-s
Avogadro's Number	6.022×10^{23} particles/mole
Charge of an Electron	1.6022×10^{-10} C
π	3.14159
e	2.718

Table 2 Index of Refraction of Common Optical Materials

Material	Index at 656.3 nm	Index at 589.2 nm	Index at 486.1 nm
Barium Flint	1.588	1.591	1.598
Borosilicate Crown, 1	1.498	1.500	1.505
Borosilicate Crown, 2	1.515	1.517	1.523
Borosilicate Crown, 3	1.509	1.511	1.517
Light Flint, 1	1.571	1.575	1.585
Light Flint, 2	1.520	1.576	1.586
Dense Flint, 2	1.612	1.617	1.629
Dense Flint, 4	1.644	1.649	1.663
Extra Dense Flint	1.456	1.458	1.463
Light Barium Crown	1.538	1.541	1.547
Quartz	1.456	1.458	1.463

Table 3 Thermal Properties of Common Metals (1 atm)

Metal	Heat of Fusion (kj/kg)	Heat of Vaporization (kj/kg)
Copper	205	4726
Gold	62.8	1701
Lead	24.7	858
Silver	105	2323
Zinc	102	1768

Table 4 Specific Heat of Common Metals (20 C)

Metal	Specific Heat (C) kj/kg-K
Copper	0.386
Gold	0.126
Lead	0.128
Silver	0.233
Zinc	0.387

Appendix B

MATHEMATICS AND TRIGONOMETRY

Trigonometry Review

The fundamental trigonometric functions are sine (sin), cosine (cos), and tangent (tan). In terms of a right triangle these are defined (using the quantities shown in Figure 1) as:

$$\sin \theta = a/c$$
$$\cos \theta = b/c$$
$$\tan \theta = b/a$$

The sides of the triangle labeled a and b are known as the legs, and the side labeled c is known as the hypotenuse.

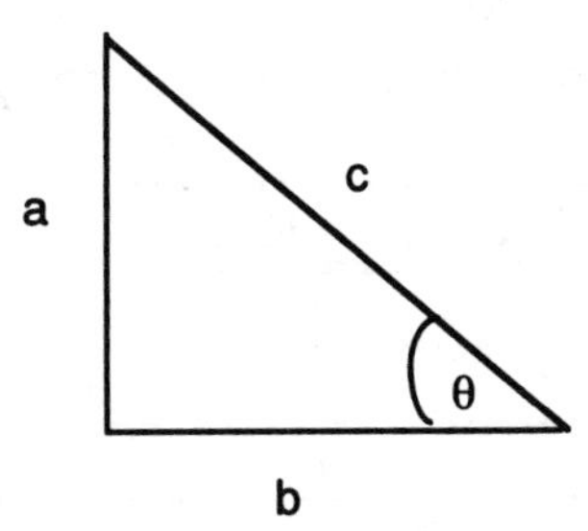

Figure 1. Right Triangle

The quantities are related to each other by the following:

$$\sin^2 \theta + \cos^2 \theta = 1$$
$$\tan \theta = (\sin \theta)/(\cos \theta)$$

Metric Prefixes		
Prefix	Symbol	Multiplier
giga	G	10^9
mega	M	10^6
kilo	k	10^3
centi	c	10^{-2}
milli	m	10^{-3}
micro	μ	10^{-6}
nano	n	10^{-9}
pico	p	10^{-12}

Scientific Notation

Scientific notation is used to express very large or very small numbers in a format that is easier to read and more simple to calculate with. To convert numbers to scientific notation, the decimal place is moved so that the number is between 1 and 10 and then a power of ten is added to produce the correct value. For example, 10,000 can be written as 10×10^3 (or 10 times 1000). As a general rule, numbers are written in scientific notation by moving the decimal point and then multiplying by a power of ten equal to the number of places the decimal point moves; positive powers when the decimal point is moved to the left and negative powers when it is moved to the right. Examine the following examples to help understand the process.

Original Number	Scientific Notation	Number of Places Moved
12,300,000	1.23×10^6	6 to the left
0.001,23	1.23×10^{-3}	3 to the right
7,08,000,000	7.08×10^8	8 to the left
0.000,403	4.03×10^{-4}	4 to the right

Appendix C

LASER SAFETY

Introduction

The principles of laser safety are generally confined to the hazards associated with the beam itself, and this appendix will be confined to these topics. However, it is important to remember that many types of lasers and applications of lasers represent associated hazards that need to be considered. Hazardous materials, fumes and especially dangerous levels of high voltage are not uncommon when dealing with lasers and should be considered when dealing with them.

The hazards of the laser beam and the appropriate safety precautions are clearly outlined and specified by the American National Standards Institute publication ANSI Z136 that is available from the Laser Institute of America. Anyone attempting significant work in the area of laser safety should make a close study of this document. There are also federal and state (in some states) laws regarding the safe use and operation of lasers which should be thoroughly understood by anyone responsible for laser safety. Appendix C summarizes the principles of laser safety and provides enough information for a working knowledge of the safe use of lasers.

Laser Beam Hazards

Laser beam hazards are described by the beam power or energy, the wavelength, the exposure time, the beam size and shape, and whether it is a reflected or direct beam (intrabeam viewing). Each of these factors is incorporated into a single value known as the Maximum Permissible Exposure (MPE) which is an indication of the maximum limit beyond which injury will occur. To understand the MPE, we need to understand the factors that affect it. The hazards of the laser beam depend on the amount of energy or power it contains. At low levels, the laser beam is hazardous to the eye and can cause severe and often permanent damage. At higher levels the beam is also a hazard to tissue in general, as well as a potential fire hazard. At any level, the reflections of the beam can also be hazardous.

Laser beam reflections are classified into three types – specular, fresnel and diffuse. The specular reflection is caused by a smooth and highly reflective surface (such as a mirror) and is generally as dangerous as the beam itself. Specular reflections contain a large percentage (usually greater than 95 %) of the original beam power and a close approximation to the beam shape.

Fresnel reflections, which come from smooth but transparent surfaces (like glass), are also hazardous but retain only a fraction (about 4 % for visible light from glass) of the original beam power. Diffuse reflections, which are from rough and opaque surfaces (like wood or unpolished metal), are least dangerous since the power levels are substantially reduced and the beam is greatly dispersed.

The dangers of the laser beam also depend on its wavelength. The human eye (see Chapter 7) transmits visible and near infrared light to the retina and absorbs ultraviolet light in the cornea, so the area of the eye that is most susceptible to damage depends on the wavelength of the beam.

The final factor associated with beam hazards is exposure duration. The amount of time tissue is exposed to a beam will affect the amount of damage that will be done. Longer durations mean more damage.

The factors affecting the MPE are determined (usually by the laser manufacturer) and the result is used to classify the laser. Laser safety classifications provide a guide to determining the potential danger a laser represents. The classifications (from least to most dangerous) are:

CLASS I. The laser beam is visible and does not exceed the MPE when viewed at minimum distance, or any laser system which cannot emit accessible radiation that exceeds the MPE.

CLASS II. Visible cw lasers not exceeding 1 mW or pulsed lasers not exceeding the exposure limit for more than .25 seconds.

CLASS IIIa. Infrared and ultraviolet lasers that cannot emit more than 0.5 W for longer than 0.25 seconds or 10 J within 0.25 seconds. Also, visible lasers that exceed the standards for Class II but cannot emit an average power of more than 0.5 W.

CLASS IIIb. Class III lasers that exceed an outpower between 1 and 5 times the Class II limits.

CLASS IV. Visible, infrared or ultraviolet lasers that exceed the maximum power or energy described in Class IIIa.

CONTROL AND SAFETY PROCEDURES

Each laser classification has controls and safety procedures associated with it. The controls include labeling, warning signs, interlocks, barriers, protective eyewear and aspects of the laser design. The safety procedures include authorization, training, limitation of access, and designation of a laser safety officer. Controls and procedures are summarized below.

PROTECTIVE HOUSING. All laser classes are required to have protective housings that prevent access and exposure to hazardous elements and emissions of the laser and accompanying system. Class IIIa, IIIb and IV lasers require interlocks on the housing which cause the laser to stop operating (including shutting down any high voltage) when the housing is removed. These interlocks are also suggested for class I and II lasers.

KEY SWITCH. Class IV lasers are required (and Class IIIb lasers are recommended) to have a master switch that is controlled by a removable key. Access to that key should be limited to qualified personnel.

BEAM PATHS AND NHZ. The path of a beam from a class IIIb or class IV laser should be enclosed or limited if feasible. If the beam path is left open, the Laser Safety Officer (see below) will establish a Nominal Hazard Zone (NHZ) where the MPE is not exceeded and within which personnel are not allowed.

EMISSION DELAY. Class IV lasers are required to have a delay between the activation of the laser and the actual emergence of the beam.

ACTIVATION WARNING SYSTEM. Class IV lasers are required to have a system that warns of the activation of the beam. The warning may be lights, and alarm or a distinctive sound that is produced when the laser is operating.

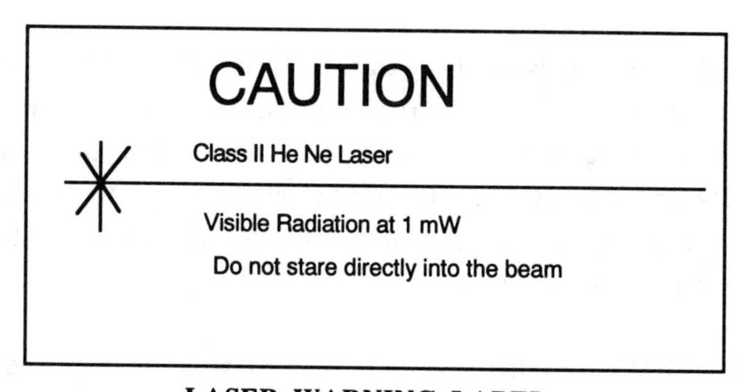

LASER WARNING LABEL

LABELS. All lasers will be labeled with their classification, precautionary instructions or protective measures, beam parameters (wavelength, power or energy) and the laser symbol (see Figure). Also, class II lasers will contain the word caution in yellow, and class III and IV lasers will contain the word danger in red. Class IIIa lasers will contain the words “avoid direct eye exposure” while class IIIb lasers will contain "avoid direct exposure to the beam" and class IV will contain "avoid eye or skin exposures to direct or scattered radiation". Non-visible lasers will include the word invisible, and all labels must be readable at a distance of two meters.

SAFETY GOGGLES. Safety goggles designed to protect the eye against the particular laser beam will be worn for all lasers above a Class II. These goggles must meet minimum standards in optical density and are available from many optics or laser supply companies.

AREA POSTINGS. Warning signs of the same design as the warning labels will be posted at each entrance to an area containing a class IIIb or class IV laser as well as in the area itself.

ENTRANCE WAY CONTROLS. Entrance ways to areas containing class IV lasers will be equipped with controls that shut down or reduce the power of the laser in the event of an unexpected entrance. If such controls limit the operation of the laser and it is evident that there is no possibility of exposure upon entrance, then the laser safety officer may allow access by properly trained personnel.

LASER SAFETY OFFICER. A laser safety officer (LSO) will be designated for institutions using class IIIb or class IV lasers. The LSO will have the authority and responsibility to monitor and enforce control of laser hazards. The LSO will also evaluate hazards, train personnel and implement appropriate engineering and procedural controls.

INDEX